Womanist AIDS Activism in the United States

Health and Aging in the Margins

Series Editor: Alexandra "Xan" C.H. Nowakowski, Florida State University

Health and Aging in the Margins expands the horizons of mainstream and academic understandings of living and aging at the intersection of diverse health experiences and marginalized biographies. Interest in life course perspectives on health and aging has expanded dramatically in recent decades. However, most attention to this topic in extant academic books has focused on more dominant social and cultural groups. This series will build on groundwork laid by these traditions to focus explicitly on the health and aging experiences of marginalized people and groups. These specific topic areas may include, but are not limited to:

Racism and People of Color	Kink Practitioners
Stigmatized Conditions	High Risk Occupations
First Generation Students	Community and Police Violence
Adoption and Donor Conception	Ethnic Discrimination
Religious and Spiritual Minorities	Asexualities
Working Class Lives	Invisible Disabilities
Unemployment	Sexism and Feminism
Intimate Partner Violence	Hate Crimes and Survivorship
Homelessness and Housing Insecurity	Food Insecurity
Rare Diseases	Sizeism and Fatphobia
Contested Disorders	Dementia and Cognitive Impairment
Social and Intellectual Differences	Communication Differences
Progressive Diseases	Childfreedom
Trans and Nonbinary Experiences	Infertility and Sterilization
Immigrant and Migrant Families	Gay / Lesbian / Bi / Pan Sexualities
Intersex Lives	Consensual Nonmonogamies
Transgender Studies	Early Mortality

The series centers ethnographic and narrative approaches to explore and understand the health and aging experiences of marginalized populations. Recruitment of authors will focus strongly on amplifying the voices of scholars who themselves have experienced intersectional marginalization, and who engage those elements of their personal biography in scholarly activity. Recent titles in the series include:

Womanist AIDS Activism in the United States: "It's Who We Are," by Angelique Harris and Omar Mushtaq

Becoming Disabled: Forging a Disability View of the World, by Jan Doolittle Wilson

Womanist AIDS Activism in the United States

"It's Who We Are"

Angelique Harris and Omar Mushtaq

LEXINGTON BOOKS
Lanham • Boulder • New York • London

Published by Lexington Books
An imprint of The Rowman & Littlefield Publishing Group, Inc.
4501 Forbes Boulevard, Suite 200, Lanham, Maryland 20706
www.rowman.com

86-90 Paul Street, London EC2A 4NE

British Library Cataloguing in Publication Information Available

Library of Congress Cataloging-in-Publication Data

Names: Harris, Angelique, author. | Mushtaq, Omar, author.
Title: Womanist AIDS activism in the United States : "it's who we are" / Angelique
    Harris and Omar Mushtaq.
Description: Lanham : Lexington Books, [2021] | Series: Health and aging in the
    margins | Includes bibliographical references and index.
Identifiers: LCCN 2021043417 (print) | LCCN 2021043418 (ebook) | ISBN
    9781793636515 (cloth ; alk. paper) | ISBN 9781793636539 (paperback) |
    ISBN 9781793636522 (ebook)
Subjects: LCSH: AIDS activists—United States. | African American women. |
    Womanism—United States. | AIDS (Disease)—Prevention—Religious aspects—
    African American churches. | AIDS (Disease)—Social aspects—United States.
Classification: LCC RA643.83 .H37 2021 (print) | LCC RA643.83 (ebook) | DDC
    362.19697/920082—dc23
LC record available at https://lccn.loc.gov/2021043417
LC ebook record available at https://lccn.loc.gov/2021043418

Contents

Chapter One

Introduction and Theoretical Framework

In her book, *In Search of Our Mothers' Gardens*, Alice Walker (1994), defines a womanist as, "a [B]lack feminist or feminist of color . . . Usually referring to outrageous, audacious, courageous or willful behavior. . . . Responsible. In charge. Serious . . . Loves the spirit . . . Loves struggle. Loves the Folk. Loves herself" (Walker 1994, xii). To Walker, feminism is a shade of womanism, just as lavender is a shade of purple. Feminism focuses on one form of inequity—gender—and the impact that it has on women. However, Walker conceptualized womanism to broaden feminism's scope of inequity because it is, "Committed to the survival and wholeness of entire people, male and female" (Walker 1994, xii). Walker believes that womanism allows individuals to rethink the ways in which women, especially Black women, interact, negotiate social and cultural demands, and engage in self and community care and activism by validating Black women's identities, experiences, empowerment, and spirituality. This book uses womanism as a theoretical framework to provide the first in-depth exploration of AIDS activism among Black women in the United States. We describe the unique ways in which race, class, gender, sexuality, and spirituality influence the experiences of Black women who are involved in AIDS activism.

Research on HIV in Black communities, and among Black women in particular, often focuses on the toll HIV has had on their lives and communities and deemphasizes Black women's active role in reducing infection rates within their communities. Previous research on Black women and activism indicated that their care for families, communities, and their overall desire for "group survival" motivates their community advocacy and social justice work (Collins 2000; Gains 1996). As such, we wanted to specifically examine how these factors, as well as their identities as Black women, played a role in their AIDS activism work and highlighted suggestions for social change

1

and transformation. Womanism serves as our theoretical framework because, as Walker explains, it provides the ideal lens to understand the impact that identity and community play in social activism among Black women.

This research is based on interviews with 36 Black women from across the United States, who engage in an array of AIDS advocacy work. This text centers the experiences of activists who have dedicated their lives to eradicating HIV from their communities. In this first chapter, we will briefly discuss feminism, intersectionality, and womanism, and explain why womanism was specifically chosen as the theoretical framework in this study. Afterward, we will discuss the study's methodological framework and study participants. Appendices A and B provide a more thorough discussion of womanism as a theoretical and methodological framework as well as detailed biographies of the 36 activists, respectively. However, first we will discuss AIDS in Black communities and previous research on Black activism and community advocacy.

AIDS IN BLACK COMMUNITIES

AIDS is one of the many negative health issues disproportionally facing Black communities. Blacks have higher rates of cancer morbidity and mortality than their White, Latinx, and Asian American/Pacific Islander counterparts (Zahnd et al. 2021). Blacks also have higher rates of high blood pressure (Rayner and Spence 2021), diabetes (Mercado et al. 2021), and heart disease (Jain et al. 2021). In addition, Black and Latinx Americans fall sick and die at disproportionally higher rates from the coronavirus (Andrasfay and Goldman 2021; Baltrus et al. 2021). However, by continuing to examine AIDS, the impact it has on Black communities, and the multiple responses to the epidemic, we can better understand—and perhaps even predict—the way health issues impact Black communities as well as community responses. As sociologist Celeste Watkins-Hayes (2014) explains, "Social status continues to play a significant role in determining who is most at risk of [HIV] infection, who is most likely to receive life-saving treatment, and how the epidemic disproportionately affects certain communities" (432).

HIV is more likely to affect Black Americans than any other racial/ethnic group in the United States (Centers for Disease Control and Prevention [CDC] 2021b; Mackenzie 2013). According to the CDC (2021b), Blacks represented approximately 13% of the total U.S. population, but accounted for 42% of new HIV infections in 2018. In that same year, Black men accounted for 31% of all new HIV infections among men and Black women accounted for 57% of women with HIV in the United States. One in 20 Black men are infected with HIV and one in 48 Black women are infected with HIV (CDC 2021b). Black men have an infection rate 6 times higher than White men and 2.5 times higher than those of Latinx men. The infection rates for Black women are 15 times higher than those of White women and 4 times higher than those of Latinx women. The CDC estimates that 22% of trans women in the U.S. are HIV-positive and 49% of trans women with HIV are Black (CDC 2021a). Additionally, many barriers including stigma (Fletcher et al., 2016), spirituality (Dalmida et al. 2012), effective case management (Halkitis et al. 2010), depression (Vyavaharkar et al. 2010), substance abuse (Wyatt et al. 2005), social support (McDoom et al. 2015), and confidentiality issues (Wyatt et al. 2005) affect Black women's access to HIV-related treatment and care.

Although men are more likely to be infected with HIV, Nancy Stoller writes, "Nothing better epitomizes the multiple voices and visions of AIDS than women's experiences of the epidemic. Here, race, class, sexuality, and gender intersect and sometimes clash" (Stoller 1998, 9). A number of factors continue to drive the high rate and disparate experiences of HIV and AIDS for different populations.

Structural Factors

Those most structurally marginalized within Black communities—e.g., gay and bisexual men, intravenous (IV) drug users, and women (both trans and cisgender)—are disproportionately affected by AIDS. A number of factors, both internal and external to Black communities, have greatly influenced HIV rates within these communities (Cohen 1999; Fullilove et al. 1990). The first is that the Black middle class and the Black Church helped construct a silence around sexuality that affected how Black communities internally responded to the AIDS crisis (Harris 2010; Cohen 1999). This homophobia and heterosexism negatively impacted efforts to combat the virus (Harris 2010; Fullilove et al. 1990). Additionally, in the early years of the epidemic, the Reagan administration cut government programs and social services for the poor and for communities of color (Stockdill 2003; Cohen 1999). Policies such as the "War on Drugs" as well as "the erosion of civil rights legislation and affirmative action, [and] the entrance of crack cocaine into U.S. cities" (Stockdill 2003, 9) further impeded responses to the epidemic in Black communities, helping to fuel HIV infection rates (Cohen 1999). In addition to public policy's impact on HIV rates, scholars have continued to highlight the impact of structural racism on individual experiences of HIV within Black communities. For example, experiences with discrimination are barriers to accessing resources that can help reduce or even prevent HIV transmission (Nydegger et al. 2021). Calabrese et al. (2014) found that medical students were less likely to prescribe a drug called pre-exposure prophylaxis (PrEP), a drug known to prevent HIV transmission, to gay and bisexual Black men since they perceived Black men as hypersexual and more likely to engage in unprotected sex. In addition, studies suggest that medical mistrust deters Black women from using PrEP because of a history of medical racism (Friedman 2009) and negative treatment from staff (Newman et al. 2008).

Research examines how sexual stereotypes negatively impact HIV transmission within Black communities and relationships (Kvasny and Payton 2018). For example, Millet et al. (2005) highlight the role of Black masculinity and the impact that the so-called "down-low culture" (heterosexual-identified men who engage in sexual behavior with other men) have on perceptions of HIV transmission within Black communities. However, literature suggests "down-low culture" arguments are empirically untrue (Bond et al. 2009; Pettaway et al. 2014). In addition, Black women in the United States are subject to respectability politics which often force them to engage in long-term or committed relationships to avoid being perceived as sexually promiscuous (French 2013; Johnson 2013). Black teenage girls who physically mature at an early age are often hypersexualized (Crooks et al. 2019) as well. Some of these teenagers internalize this hypersexualization and were consequently more likely to engage in sexual activity at an earlier age (Townsend et al. 2010; Stephens and Phillips 2005). As a result, Black sexuality—among men, women, and children—is further eroticized and stigmatized because these analyses ignore not only the role of structural racism, but how other racial/ethnic groups engage in similar sexual and/or potentially risk-taking behaviors (Saleh and Operario 2009).

Black Women and AIDS Activism

Black women have consistently provided leadership and support to their communities in the struggle against AIDS since the start of the epidemic (McLane-Davison 2016). Women's infection rates were relatively overshadowed by their male counterparts, and, as such, AIDS interventions and research on experiences with the virus largely focused on men (Patton 2005; Corea 1992). However, as Black women are disproportionately impacted by HIV, a significant body of research began to emerge that focuses on their specific experiences (Campbell and Soeken 1999; Fullilove et al. 1990). Much of this work primarily concentrated on their risk factors and the impact HIV has had on their lives (Berger 2010; Ingram and Hutchinson 2000), such as the negative impact that HIV criminalization laws have on Black women (Tharao et al 2013). Nonetheless, Black women have played a major role in the organization of specific health initiatives to promote AIDS awareness and education (McLane-Davidson 2016; Harris 2010). For example, Black women have founded AIDS campaigns and organizations such as The Balm in Gilead, The Well Project, Black AIDS Institute, The Positive Women's Network, and Sister Love. However, considering the leadership role that Black women have taken in AIDS discourse, particularly within Black communities, few studies (Harris 2010; Reeder et al. 2001) specifically examine AIDS activism and advocacy within Black communities.

Research on AIDS and racial disparities consists of studies that examine the high rates of HIV and AIDS among Black women in the United States and abroad (Brijnath 2007; Whitmore et al. 2005). Research also examines AIDS in Black communities (Cohen 1999; Dalton 1989), issues pertaining to sexuality (Hoosen and Collins 2004; Sweet and Jemmott 1991), and the influence of AIDS stigma (Herek and Capitanio 1999) on the lives of women of color with AIDS (Berger 2010).

Scholarship on AIDS activism examines the intersections that race, class, gender, and sexuality have on AIDS activism discourse (Stockdill 2003; Stoller 1998). Research explores AIDS activism among women overall (The ACT UP/NY Women and AIDS Book Group 1990), within Black communities (Cohen 1999), and within the Black Church (Harris 2010). Research examines the motivations behind AIDS activism in Black communities in the U.S. (Reeder et al. 2001) and activism among Black women in sub-Saharan Africa (Robins 2006). Social work scholar Denise McLane-Davison's sole (2016; 2018) and coauthored (Reeder et al. 2001) works do specifically examine the leadership roles Black women have taken in addressing AIDS in Black communities. Using a Black feminist analysis, McLane-Davison (2016) examines the ways in which a group of Black women have taken on leadership roles in the fight against AIDS. However, this current study provides a more nuanced discussion of AIDS activism and advocacy work within Black communities, and, importantly, explores womanism as a framework through which to examine activism, advocacy, and overall sociopolitical involvement among Black women.

FEMINISM, BLACK FEMINISM, INTERSECTIONALITY, AND WOMANISM

Social movement theorists argue that structurally marginalized groups, such as Black women, have a unique perspective of social change and justice because of their relative lack of institutionalized power and access to resources (Chun et al. 2013; Cho et al. 2013). Structurally marginalized identities and their intersections result in unique lived experiences and world views. Since

Sojourner Truth, Black feminists and intersectionality scholars and activists have complicated notions of single-identity issues that traditional feminists have often employed, by emphasizing that not only is there no hierarchy of identity and oppression (Lorde 1984a; hooks 1981), but that identities intersect to form unique issues and experiences of oppression. Feminism, Black feminism, intersectionality, and womanism are theoretical frameworks that attempt to understand the sociocultural factors that influence gender-based inequities; yet, their approaches are vastly different. Here, we define feminism, Black feminism, intersectionality, and womanism:

Feminism: a theoretical analysis of gender inequalities and the advocacy and promotion of women's rights and inclusion.

Black Feminism: a theoretical framework and body of knowledge that centers the voices, experiences, lives, and oppressions of Black women.

Intersectionality: an analytical tool which examines the ways in which social identities, such as race, class, gender, and sexuality intersect to inform the lives, experiences, and oppressions of people.

Womanism: a theoretical framework and worldview that conjoins notions of identity, spirituality, and social justice. Similar to intersectionality, womanism examines the intersections of identity: however, it emphasizes how spirituality, the pursuit of social justice, and the responsibility of community support is an integral part of one's activist identity. Although informed by the experiences of women of color, womanism is not gender specific.

In order to understand how Black women mobilize against AIDS, we apply a womanist framework. As discussed above, Walker (1994, xii) notes that "womanism is to feminism as lavender is to purple;" as such, womanism can also be viewed as a response to feminism. First- and second-wave feminism focused on attaining equal rights for women, but these movements were broadly framed around White middle-class women and overlooked the struggles of Black women. Womanism and Black feminism addressed these gaps by centering Black women's experiences, while also highlighting racism, classism, heterosexism, and other inequities. In order to address these inequities, these frameworks deploy intersectionality as a tool to develop their epistemologies and encourage mobilization. This section will provide a brief introduction to womanism as a framework. It will describe womanism and Black feminism, as well as examine how intersectionality augments these frameworks.

To preface our conversation, we realize that womanism, Black feminism, and intersectionality have rich bodies of literature. As such, we will further elaborate on the nuances of womanism, Black feminism, and intersectionality, especially in regard to womanism's relationship with Black feminism and intersectionality. Indeed, other scholars, such as Collins (1996; 2002), have engaged in these discussions at length. However, to focus our conversation around the application of womanism, we briefly provide an abridged version of this conversation.

Womanism as a Theoretical Framework

The main theoretical crux of our analysis is womanism. Based on Walker's definition of womanism, we highlight three main dimensions of womanism: empowerment, community centrism, and social justice.

1. Womanism as Empowerment

Womanism stresses Black women's empowerment. With its emphasis on self-love and self-acceptance, womanism acknowledges that Black women endure both structural and institutional marginalization. According to Walker (1994, xii), Black women counter their oppression because they "take charge" and embody "strength."

2. Womanism and Community Centrism

Womanism centers the needs of the community. As mentioned above, womanists are "committed to survival and wholeness of entire people, male and female" (Walker 1994, xii). American womanism's commitment parallels its Africana counterpart (Hudson-Weems 2019), where collectivistic notions of "wholeness" and "unity" drive Black women's community engagement.

3. Womanism and Social Justice

Womanist politics focus on Black women's desire for social change. In addition to ending the oppression that *Black women* face, womanism focuses on a universalist ethos that focuses on ending *all* oppression for *everyone*.

Given these three dimensions of womanism, our analysis centers womanism, as throughout our analysis we found that the respondents emphasized their own agency in AIDS activism (empowerment), emphasized their communities (community centrism), and focused on dismantling all structures of social inequities, including classism, racism, sexism, and homophobia (social justice).

Black Feminism as a Part of Womanism

As theoretical and methodical frameworks, womanism and Black feminism are in dialogue with one another, and, indeed, several points highlight how Black feminism is part of womanist epistemology. First, both womanism and Black feminism center Black women's experiences. Additionally, since womanism focuses on empowerment, Black feminist scholars, such as Audre Lorde and bell hooks, have written extensively on White supremacy, sexism, homophobia, and other structures that have negatively impacted Black women and how they resist these structures. Furthermore, Black feminism addresses gaps in White-dominated epistemology; as Patricia Hill Collins (2002) describes, the knowledge production process ignores Black women's experiences. Womanism highlights the idea of centering Black women's everyday experiences as its epistemology, including Black women's emphasis on their communities. Finally, Black feminism focuses on equal rights for women and men globally, as womanism preaches a universality politic that bases its ethic of liberation for everyone (Collins 1996).

Intersectionality Is a Tool of Black Feminism and Womanism

When asked to speak during the 1851 women's rights convention in Akron, Ohio, abolitionist Sojourner Truth proclaimed, "Ain't I a Woman?" in an effort to describe challenges unique to Black women and explain the interconnectedness of the racism and sexism she experienced. In 1989, Black legal scholar Kimberlé Williams Crenshaw, the founder of the "Say Her Name" campaign (Khaleeli 2021)—a campaign designed to bring attention to the Black women who have been murdered by police—coined the term "intersectionality," (Harris and Bartlow 2015) which Black feminist scholar Patricia Hill Collins (2000) would later describe as the "analysis claiming that systems of race, social class, gender, sexuality, ethnicity, nation, and age form mutually constructing features of social organization which shape Black women's experiences, and, in turn, are shaped by Black women" (299). In essence, intersectionality argues that multiple systems of inequities impact Black women, and, importantly, informs their worldviews and social interactions.

Although intersectionality was first used as a framework to examine Black women and how intersecting oppressions impact their lives and experiences, this framework was expanded to include the experiences of other groups with structurally marginalized identities (Choo and Ferree 2010). Scholars Cho, Crenshaw, and McCall argue that intersectionality has expanded to a field of study to include, "investigation[s] of intersectional dynamics . . . debates about the scope and content of intersectionality as a theoretical and methodological paradigm, and . . . political interventions employing an intersectional lens" (2013, 785). Intersectional frameworks have often been applied to examine identity, encourage activism to reduce oppression, and address social ills among structurally marginalized groups (Chun et al. 2013).

Intersectionality overlaps with Black feminism and womanism in several ways. First, intersectionality focuses on a "matrix of oppression" (Collins 2002) and highlights how one's experience is shaped by multiple structures. For example, Black women navigate experiences of racism, sexism, and misogynoir. While not comparable to Black women's oppression, Black men likewise navigate racism and a type of gender-based discrimination (Assari 2017; Assari et al. 2017); however they also experience gender-based privilege. Womanism and Black feminism utilize intersectional frameworks as they both emphasize the ways in which intersecting identities impact the experiences of Black women, but from slightly different perspectives. Womanism highlights Black women's experiences as a source of strength and empowerment. Similarly, Black feminism highlights the experiences of Black women as they navigate sexism and racism. As such, womanism and Black feminism apply the notion that Black women inhabit specific intersecting identities and navigate multiple structures of domination.

Additionally, as mentioned earlier, womanism and Black feminism apply intersectionality's notion that it is an epistemology that centers Black women. Collins (2002) describes how intersectionality enables Black feminism to address how Black women's experiences are overlooked in academic literature and methodologies. For example, Collins (2002, 253) writes,

> *In general, scholars, publishers, and other experts represent specific interests and credentialing processes, and their knowledge claims must satisfy the political and epistemological criteria of the contexts in which they reside . . . [knowledge generation] is controlled by elite White men, knowledge validation processes reflect this group's interests. Although designed to represent and protect the interests of powerful White men, neither schools, government, the media and other social institutions that house these processes nor the actual epistemologies that they promote need be managed by White men themselves.*

While Collins highlights how knowledge is dominated by White men, she provides an example by addressing a specific instance in which mainstream epistemology negates Black women's experiences: "Individual African-American women's narratives about being single mothers are often rendered invisible in quantitative research methodologies that erase individuality in favor of proving patterns of welfare abuse" (Collins 2002, 255). On this epistemological and methodological note, she explains, "For most African-American women those individuals who have lived through the experiences about which they claim to be experts are more believable and credible than those who have merely read or thought about such experiences. Thus, lived experience as a criterion for credibility frequently is invoked by U.S. Black women when making knowledge claims" (Collins 2002, 258). Similar to this thought, womanism also highlights Black women's epistemology and suggests that storytelling is a key aspect of how Black women can develop their epistemology. Thus, by privileging how Black women generate knowledge, Black feminism and intersectionality affirm Black women's experiences as a means of generating both academic and lived epistemologies.

Additionally, Black feminism and womanism deploy intersectionality as a means of empowerment. By highlighting Black women's unique subject position as individuals who suffer from racial and gendered discrimination, intersectionality provides the framework to help Black women identify common issues, mobilize, and engage in activism. For example, Black feminism focuses on Black women's experiences with White supremacy and sexism, and, ultimately, influences social movements, such as Black Lives Matter and Black Trans Lives Matter. These movements center both Black women's experiences and their communities. While Black feminism influences social movements, womanism explicitly describes how Black women's circumstances empower them to challenge social inequities.

Addressing Black Feminism and Intersectionality's Limitations

When applied to AIDS scholarship, some researchers use intersectionality as a theoretical framework to understand gender dynamics more broadly (Dworkin et al. 2006), while others document how Black men negotiate poverty, incarceration, racial discrimination, and other forms of social inequity (Bowleg et al. 2014). Gender studies scholar Michele Tracy Berger argues that AIDS should be examined using an intersectional framework and uses the term "intersectional stigma" (24) to describe the unique experiences that Black women face based on the intersections of their race, class, gender, and sexual identities in conjunction with a stigmatized health issue, such as HIV. As Watkins-Hayes (2014) contends, "Unlike many other illnesses, [AIDS] has a particular cultural significance that obliges its carriers, and those most intimately involved in their lives, to grapple with weighty and contentious social issues: sex, sexuality, drugs, class, race, gender, and inequality of exposure to harm" (432). While intersectionality has been applied to AIDS research, the framework has limitations.

As will be discussed in more detail in this book, our respondents explained how race and other factors were important parts of their identity and identity development beyond solely their gender identity. Black women and other women of color have long criticized dominant feminist paradigms for not addressing concerns facing all women, particularly women of color, such as the racial and class oppressions they often experience (Collins 2000). Womanism provides a more nuanced analysis, for, "Unlike feminism, and despite its name, womanism does not emphasize or privilege gender or sexism, rather it elevates all sites and forms of oppression, whether they are based on social-address categories like gender, race, or class, to a level of equal concern and action" (Phillips 2006, xx). Although Black feminist theory can be used to address the experiences of women of color, in general, it explicitly privileges the experiences of Black women (Collins 2000; 2002). Intersectional frameworks within Black feminist theory have been applied to the experiences of other women of color (Choo and Ferree 2010); however, in her development of womanism, Walker specifically argues that womanism is a framework that emphasizes the experiences of all structurally marginalized groups, including Black women, men of color, and non-Black women of color (Walker 1994). Nonetheless, womanism has primarily been embraced by Black women throughout the African diaspora. At its core, womanism emphasizes identity, experiences, and the role individuals have in advocacy and enacting social change.

Womanism and Social Change

Womanism is both a theoretical perspective and a "worldview" used by international scholars to explain how intersecting oppressions shape the perspective of women of color, and in turn, this worldview influences Black women's desire for social justice (Phillips 2006). Womanist scholar Layli Phillips (2006) writes,

> *Womanism is a social change perspective rooted in Black women's and other women of color's everyday experiences and everyday methods of problem solving in everyday spaces, extended to the problem of ending all forms of oppression for all people, restoring the balance between people and the environment/ nature, and reconciling human life with the spiritual dimension. (xx)*

Here, Phillips posits the notion that womanism is more than an analytic framework; it is a framework for "social change." Phillips advocates a practical approach for ending social inequities and highlights a spiritual dimension to eradicating social injustice. In comparison to Black feminist thought, Duran (2010) argues "womanism may be defined as a Black feminist view that is community-orientated as opposed to the sort of feminist view that has the privilege and luxury of defining oppression in terms of male dominance" (175). Although we highlighted how the intersectional perspective argued by Black feminism is similar to womanism (Collins 1996), compared to womanism, Black feminism underemphasizes how intersectional oppression is framed in the context of the pursuit of social justice and informs Black women's identities.

Unlike intersectionality, which was primarily developed and used as analytical and methodological tool for academics to understand oppression and eventually leaked into mainstream discourse as a descriptive and explanatory term for Black women's oppression, womanism is a system of values and norms that shape Black women's experiences and their realities. Put another way, though intersectionality has been deployed as a tool to shape social movements and understandings of misogynoir in America, intersectionality is the "theory" of Black women's experiences, whereas womanism is the theory, belief, and practice. Additionally, womanism is both social justice-orientated and spiritually orientated, as womanist scholars have argued for increased attention to the spiritual lives of women of color (Black women in particular), and how spirituality shapes their decisions and identities and motivates their social justice activities (Brown and Brown 2003). Furthermore, womanism and intersectionality differ as womanism is rooted in Afrocentric notions of group survival and care, while intersectionality is much more focused on the individual, their care, and their interactions (Dandridge 2004).

As such, we focus on womanism as our framework instead of intersectionality because intersectionality is primarily used as an analytical framework as opposed to serving as a meaningful worldview. Second, although intersectionality has been used to inform activism, it does not highlight how activism is an integral part of one's identity.

Women of color, especially Black women, have critiqued feminism for not addressing concerns facing all women, and the race-based and class-based oppressions they often experience (Collins 2000). Somewhat akin to Black feminist theory, womanism argues that racism, sexism, and class discrimination intersect to create a unique form of oppression. Black feminist thought also explicitly discusses the importance of social justice and community activism among Black women. However, although researchers apply Black feminist theory to address the experiences of women of color, in general, it explicitly privileges the experiences of Black women more specifically (Collins 2000; 2002).

Womanism more clearly emphasizes the essential role that people can play in their own survival and the support they provide their communities. Rita Dandridge (2004, 10) argues that "womanism identifies the Africana [Black women of African descent] woman as doer, the agent implementing communal wholeness. As an activist, she fights for the care and protection of others and the recognition and naming for herself as 'woman.'" Compared to intersectionality, womanism provides a more focused understanding of how women with intersecting identities understand their own social justice activism.

STUDY METHODOLOGY

This book applies a womanist framework to examine activism among Black women. We explore one principal question: What encourages AIDS activism among Black women? To answer this question, our project examines a purposive sample of 36 Black women AIDS activists via snowball sampling techniques (Seidman 2006) and a recruitment advertisement.

The respondents consisted of cisgender Black women who identify themselves as AIDS activists. These study participants engaged in paid and unpaid AIDS activism work on their own, or through AIDS service organizations, churches, and other health-based organizations throughout the United States. They also provided AIDS advocacy and education to their respective communities through various community outreach efforts. After IRB approval was first obtained, which detailed procedures that guaranteed our respondents confidentiality and anonymity, a pilot study was originally conducted with the first 10 respondents to examine the feasibility of the recruitment methods as well as to develop future research questions to further construct the theory for analysis. Once the recruitment method and interview questions were assessed, the original IRB application was revised and approved, and an additional 26 respondents were recruited as part of this study.

The initial recruitment goal was to obtain a purposive sample of at least 30 Black women AIDS activists who worked within four geographic regions throughout the United States: the Northeast, South, Midwest, and West Coast. This geographic breakdown provided a deeper understanding of the regional variables that may influence the respondents' activism work. Our goal was to get a minimum of six interviews per geographic region. We oversampled in the Northeast and the South because these regions have the highest rates of HIV and the largest concentration of Blacks in the nation. The number 30 was selected as previous research indicates that saturation occurs (respondents begin to report similar stories) within the initial 12 interviews and can begin to occur with as few as six interviews (Guest et al. 2006). Due to oversampling in the Northeast and the South, the final total resulted in 36 study participants.

The activists who participated in this sample were admitted based on their racial and gender identification; their level of engagement in AIDS education, prevention, and intervention work targeting structurally marginalized groups (primarily women and gay and bisexual men); and the length of time in which they were engaged in AIDS activism work. Only respondents who have worked in AIDS activism for five years or more were recruited as this would better help us assess the impact that their activism has had on their identity (and vice versa) over time.

In order to obtain a diverse sample, subjects who represented a wide array of AIDS activism work were contacted. Researchers initiated contact and requested interviews with 11 respondents. An additional 25 respondents were recruited via an advertisement posted on the National Black Women's HIV/AIDS Network's Facebook page. Subjects who fulfilled the criteria described above were identified and contacted via email. This introductory email described the reasons why they were selected to participate in the study and each email was followed up with a phone call to the respondent's home or office. All study participants agreed to participate in the project upon the initial email or phone call. Once respondents agreed to participate, a date and time for the interview was set.

A majority of the interviews were conducted over the telephone (34) and two were conducted in person. One in-person interview was conducted at the home of the respondent and the other was conducted in the respondent's office. Phone interviews were primarily used for the convenience of both the respondent and researcher, and in order to save time and money. Telephone interviews were also conducted as part of the initial pilot study to assess the feasibility of conducting telephone interviews for this project. Although research indicates that there are some disadvantages with telephone interviewing (lower response rates and respondents feeling uncomfortable answering sensitive questions over the phone), this research has shown that the advantages (lower research costs, more control over situational variables, and easier ability to code and analyze the data) outweigh the disadvantages (Gillham 2005). Researchers have found that in some cases, data collection is enhanced by telephone interviewing (Gillham 2005). Likewise, there was a significantly higher response rate considering the subjects opted to be interviewed over the telephone instead of being interviewed in person. Neither the breadth nor depth of the telephone interviews differed substantially from those conducted in person. As such, telephone interviewing was deemed an acceptable method for data collection for this project.

Consent was obtained in writing for interviews conducted in person and verbally for those conducted over the telephone. All but two respondents waived their right to anonymity and some even encouraged the use of their real names. However, we applied pseudonyms in lieu of the respondents' real names in order to protect the identities of our respondents. Detailed biographies of the study participants are located in Appendix B.

Interview questions included but were not limited to: their discussions on their identities, their religious and spiritual beliefs, their perceptions and reasons for their own activism, their AIDS outreach activities, as well as their demographic information. Since this is the first study of its kind, concentration was placed on inductively generating theoretical propositions using a "grounded" theory approach (Charmaz 2002; Glaser and Strauss 2017). Interviews were recorded using a digital voice recorder and were subsequently uploaded and transcribed on a computer. All of the interviews received a line-by-line analysis and were coded based on themes or concepts (Charmaz 2002). As themes began to emerge, we applied womanism as a theoretical and analytical framework to expand understandings of the social and cultural conditions that encourage AIDS activism among the respondents. A more comprehensive analysis of womanism as a theoretical and methodological framework is found in Appendix A.

Interviews ranged in length from 40 minutes to three hours and 28 minutes. Interviews averaged one hour and 46 minutes. A little over 65 interview hours were recorded. All of the activists self-identified as Black women. We did not inquire as to whether or not our participants identified as cisgender women as it was not relevant to the current study (in future analyses, it would be important to examine how Black trans women, specifically, engage in AIDS activism). Respondents lived and worked within the four geographic regions of the United States (the Northeast, South, Midwest, and West Coast) identified for this study. As stated above, our initial goal was to attempt to obtain a minimum of six interviews per geographic region using snowball sampling techniques. Although we fell short of our initial recruitment goal of six respondents per geographic region, we were able to recruit significantly more respondents in the Northeast than originally planned. The geographic breakdown of the respondents are as follows: Northeast N=18 (locations include Boston, Philadelphia, New York City, and smaller communities in Upstate New York); the South N=9 (locations include Washington DC, Maryland, smaller communities in North and South Carolina, Dallas, Baton Rouge, and New Orleans); the West Coast N=5 (locations include Los Angeles, Oakland, and San Diego); and the Midwest N=4 (locations include Denver, Detroit, and Milwaukee).

All but one respondent (who was born in Haiti but raised in the U.S. since she was 5) were born in the U.S. and all respondents had worked in AIDS activism for at least five years at the time of the interview. Respondents ranged in age from 30–65. All of the respondents had at least a high school education. Most respondents had a college degree, and half had a post-graduate degree. At the time of the interview, all but two respondents either worked or volunteered for AIDS service agencies. These women defined their activism as media and street activism, peer education, advocacy, and leadership. All of the respondents indicated that although they wanted to help *all* people living with AIDS and prevent new infections among all people, regardless of their sexual orientation, racial/ethnic group, or gender, Blacks (Black women in particular), were the primary target of their activism efforts. In terms of their sexuality, most women identified as heterosexual and seven women identified as queer (defined as any sexual orientation that was not heterosexual). One woman chose to not to disclose her sexual orientation. It is important to note that the HIV status of the activists was not a subject of inquiry for this project, and as such, questions were not asked about their HIV status. Nonetheless, all respondents indicated whether or not they were HIV-positive during the course of the interview, particularly when we discussed the motivations behind their activism.

Reflexivity

As qualitative researchers, we acknowledge that our social positions impact our understandings of the theoretical frameworks, the data collection, and the data analysis process. Additionally, we acknowledge our positionality as researchers and our varying degrees of insider/outsider access to this project. Thus, while we acknowledge how our social positions might have impacted our project, we largely focus our efforts on conducting an empirical study, where the analysis largely relied on systematically evaluating data in an attempt to offset bias as opposed to centering our identities as the means of inquiry. Along this vein, our conclusions about womanism, Black feminism, and intersectionality are based on the data and the patterns that emerged from the data as theory emerges from the data in many forms of qualitative research. In other words, while we acknowledge that our understandings of womanism and Black feminism affected data collection (i.e., interview instrument) and data analysis, our conclusions about the theory are based on patterns found within the data itself. Additionally, while we acknowledge the contributions of interdisciplinary work that focus on Black women, we focus our discussion around womanist, Black feminist, and sociological literature. We emphasize that this process of attempting to divorce our positionalities from the project is far from perfect.

In pursuit of centering Black women's voices and narratives, a positivistic framework can indeed be problematic from the perspective of anti-positivistic scholarship. However, Collins (2002, 256) asserts that at times, positivism can be deployed strategically, especially when trying to dismantle White supremacist epistemologies: "However, they [Black women scholars] simultaneously needed to challenge the same structure that granted them legitimacy. Their responses to this dilemma reflect the strategic use of the tools of positivism when needed, coupled with overt challenges to positivism when that seemed feasible . . ." While we recognize that, as Audre Lorde (1984b) asserts, "the master's tools will never dismantle the master's house," we choose to be transparent about our epistemology in our attempt to center Black women's voices and epistemologies.

BOOK LAYOUT

This book focuses on religion, spirituality, emotions, and identity in Black women's AIDS activism. In this first chapter, we reviewed literature on AIDS in Black communities and womanism as a theoretical framework. We explained how Black communities are negatively impacted by HIV and AIDS due to a variety of social inequities. We also applied Black feminist, intersectional, and womanist frameworks to address how Black communities mobilize against these social inequities, including HIV and AIDS.

Chapter 2 focuses on race and gender identity among our study participants and highlights the importance that their AIDS advocacy and community work have on their identity and sense of self. In this chapter, we explore how Black women have been at the forefront of mobilizing their communities, and how cultural expectations influence their mobilization efforts. While our findings mirror these patterns, we also find Black women disidentify with mainstream feminism because feminism typically focuses its analysis on gender disparities and ignores conversations around race and class. We discuss these findings in more detail in that chapter.

Chapter 3 explores religion and spirituality and the role they play in Black lives and communities, and, in particular, how they impact the activism work of the women in our study. While the literature discusses the importance of religiosity in Black communities, we find that the women in our study have had negative experiences with many Black churches because of perceived homophobia and sexism. We demonstrate how these experiences lead our respondents to distinguish religiosity from spirituality in their lives.

Chapter 4 considers how emotions help motivate the women in our study, and how they motivate activists in general, to enact social change. We examine how social movement literature addresses the intersection of race and gender in their analyses of emotion and feeling. We find that Black women are influenced by the love they feel for their communities, the pain of losing their loved ones, and the solidarity they feel with one another.

Chapter 5 explores conceptualizations of AIDS information and knowledge among these activists and how they work to address gaps in AIDS knowledge. We review literature that explores education around HIV and AIDS prevention and disparities within Black communities. We then address how these women posit suggestions for social change within their own communities.

Chapter 6 concludes the book with a discussion of the theoretical contributions of our research on womanism, studies of activism among Black women and women of color, and social movement theory. As previously mentioned, in Appendix A we have included a more detailed discussion of womanism as a theoretical and methodical framework. Appendix B provides detailed biographies of all 36 activists interviewed in this study.

Chapter Two

Identity and Social Justice

Anthropologist and author Zora Neale Hurston describes Black women as "de mule uh de world" (Hurston 1937, 14). In her seminal work, *Their Eyes Were Watching God*, Hurston implies that Black women are oppressed, burdened, and are responsible for working to support and provide care for not only their families, but also their communities. Although met with mixed reviews when Hurston's novel was published in 1937, it gained in popularity decades after Hurston's death, with the help of prominent Black scholars and activists, including Alice Walker, who tracked down Hurston's unmarked grave to honor her with a tombstone. In her work, Hurston highlights not only how Black women are oppressed, but also how they strive for liberation.

Black women have a history of quickly mobilizing to address community concerns, particularly concerns around inequities (Giddens 1996; White 1999). For Black women, activism is not individually focused, and their "visions are not limited to a narrow and essentialist identity politics" (Sudbury 2005). This has led Black women to be at the forefront of social justice movements for Blacks in America, ranging from the abolitionist movement to Black Lives Matter (Garza 2016). Writers and activists (Wells 2002; Collins 2000) have long recognized the gender, racial, class, and sexual oppressions that Black women have historically experienced and the impact these oppressions have on their community work and activism (Giddens 1996; Springer 2005). In an attempt to address inequities, feminist perspectives have attempted to explain how and why women mobilize; however, as mentioned in the previous chapter, Black women have also been alienated by feminist politics that have largely served White, middle-class women (Zinn and Dill 2016). In this chapter, we explore the impact that activism and advocacy have on the self-perceptions of Black women as community "caretakers" and how these perceptions influence their identities as Black women and as activists.

FEMINISM AND BLACK WOMEN

Feminism is both an epistemology and political movement that focuses on women's rights (Collins 1996). While both feminist theory and practice focus on understanding gender inequities between women and men, feminist *theory* focuses on women (and gendered minorities) as an oppressed subject within a patriarchal structure, whereas feminist *politics* focuses on organizing and social movements around attaining equal rights for women and gendered minorities (Collins 2000). Western feminist theory and praxis developed in "waves." With figures like Susan B. Anthony and Elizabeth Cady Stanton, first-wave feminism focused mainly on women's property and voting rights. Once these rights were attained, second-wave feminism focused on attaining legal protections within the public sphere. For example, second-wave feminism included marshaling women away from the home and into the workplace, gender parity laws, reproductive rights, and sexual harassment protections. Third-wave feminism began to address intersections of gendered experiences—e.g., women, of color rights, queer rights, and trans rights. Although an activist during the first wave of feminism, Sojourner Truth's focus on the experiences of Black women and more intersectional analyses of gendered experiences did not become part of widespread discussions in feminism until the third wave.

While feminism continues its decades-long attempts to broaden its scope to become more inclusive, feminism, which is also often known as Western feminism or White feminism (Hawkesworth 2012), has its limitations. Feminism often frames issues around White, middle-class, heterosexual women, and has alienated women from structurally marginalized backgrounds, including Black women (Davis 1981). For example, feminist scholar Nancy Hoffman (1986, 2) writes, "A more typical activist was Elizabeth Cady Stanton, who, spurred to organize for women's rights by her experience with the anti-feminism of abolitionists, focused her attention largely on the legal and domestic problems of educated [W]hite women. To dramatize women's powerlessness, she frequently made an analogy between slavery and women's oppression." Interestingly, later feminist theorical scholarship drew similar analogies (Simons 1979).

This pattern of framing feminism as a White, middle-class movement continued onward in the 1950s through the 1980s (Zinn and Dill 2016), during which multiple struggles were defined by the needs of White women. For example, Friedan's (2010) *The Feminine Mystique* critiqued women's cult of domesticity, but this "cult" largely applied to White, middle-class women. Feminism's White dominance also occurred in reproductive rights, where White women were fighting for the right to have reproductive autonomy, whereas Black and Latinx women were being forcibly sterilized (Roberts

1999; Washington 2006). Additionally, while Whiteness heavily permeated feminist priorities, it also made Black women's contributions and leadership invisible. For example, decades before Hillary Rodham Clinton, Congresswoman Shirley Chisolm was the first woman to pursue a nomination for U.S. President from a major political party, and it was Black women who initiated some of the first sexual harassment lawsuits in the U.S. (The Nation 2017). Continuously, White feminism glossed over issues that were important to women of color, including Black women's economic interests (Torrey 1979) and labor inequities (Dill 1979). In addition to its issues around race, White feminism was inherently heterosexist, overlooking the issues and concerns of lesbians and women in same-gender-loving relationships (Lorde 1984a). Thus, feminism has historically alienated Black women and their communities.

ACTIVISM AMONG BLACK WOMEN AND COMMUNITY SUPPORT

Black women have always been charged with caring and fighting for the survival and well-being of their children, families, loved ones, and communities (Collins 2000; Gilkes 1980). What Collins refers to as this "othermothering" is, in essence, the location where caregiving, motherhood, and social justice intersect. Collins explains,

> *Community "othermothers" participation in activist mothering demonstrates a clear rejection of separateness and individual interest as the basis of either community organization or individual self-actualization. Instead, the connectedness with others and common interest expressed by community othermothers model a very different value system, one whereby ethics of caring and personal accountability move communities forward.* (191–192)

As such, there is a cultural expectation to promote social change and engage in community work which is vital to Black culture and Black advancement (Gilkes 2001; McDonald 1997). For many Black women, the focus on community care is a cultural expectation and integral to their sense of identity (Collins 2000; Gilkes 2001).

Our 36 respondents described how their activism centered around social justice and community service. They explained that AIDS devastated their communities and they wanted to, as Rose, a 42-year-old documentary filmmaker, stated, "give back" to their communities. Likewise, Alyssa, who worked in HIV prevention for eight years, said that she saw herself in the women she helps and noted, "I'm in the age bracket, between 24 and 35, where the statistic of me becoming infected is like within a pin drop." The activists emphasized that AIDS was among the many social issues impacting Black communities. Glenda, who worked in AIDS activism for over 18 years at a major AIDS service organization targeting Blacks in New York City, explained that there were "bigger political, social, economic issues that we all knew were driving the epidemic." In particular, participants described the relationship AIDS has to community issues and concerns around social justice and overall group survival.

Community Issues

Respondents discussed the many social justice issues—e.g., incarceration, poverty, and drug abuse—that are interrelated and are fueling the AIDS epidemic in Black communities. Forty-one-year-old, Los Angeles-based AIDS advocate Isabella explained that in order to address AIDS in Black communities, one must first:

Address the underlying issue, and the underlying issue is if you have high unemployment and you have high substance abuse and alcoholism, that puts people at risk. Meaning if you're unemployed, you're thinking about you might be depressed, and if you're depressed, the way that you cope with it—some people—is that they use alcohol or drugs. Then on top of that, if you have mass incarceration of a population, then for the women, they're dealing with concurrent relationships. So, their main man is incarcerated, but they may feel that they need to have another relationship in order to get their needs met. So, I think by having those social injustices that's brought on, I think it will drive an epidemic in our community.

Similarly, Dana, a 59-year-old activist who worked for a Philadelphia AIDS service organization, remarked,

Well, I think it's economic justice or economic injustice. We always say that HIV is not just a virus. HIV is part of social and economic inequality. So, when we started talking about HIV prevention justice, we had to describe it. And we were talking about systems beyond your control that makes you vulnerable for HIV . . . just where you live makes you more vulnerable to HIV because the pool of partners is already infected.

The women in our study gave a variety of reasons for the escalating HIV rates within Black communities, including Isabella's account of the impact of substance abuse and incarceration on Black women, whereas Dana described how economic justice affects one's vulnerability to AIDS. Similarly, they understood that these issues would have to be addressed within Black communities before AIDS can be completely eradicated in Black communities.

Glenda explained that AIDS "highlighted the unfairness, disparity, racism, [and] sexism . . . [as well as] psychosocial, economic, societal issues. . . . We've got to end all of those things so that we can end HIV/AIDS." By noting the multidimensional nature of the AIDS epidemic, Glenda also noted the multiple factors that explain the epidemic's impact on Black communities. The women in our study believe that the primary reasons for the escalating rates of HIV in Black communities include, as Jocelyn, a 51-year-old activist from New York City articulated during our interview, "poverty, racism, gender, and equality, and attach religious and cultural barriers . . . Christianity and Muslim religions makes it very hard to negotiate safer sex."

The respondents were aware of how multiple social issues impacted one's experience. As described by the women, economic, social, and religious factors impeded HIV prevention efforts. As Stockdill (2003) and Watkins-Hayes (2014) note, multiple structures of social inequities, such as economic barriers, affect one's vulnerability to the AIDS virus. While the respondents described how these broader factors impact Black communities, as echoed by Broaddus et al. (2015), some respondents described the importance of negotiating safer sex and interpersonal agency. As a result, activists were aware of how their fight for survival is impacted by multiple systems of social inequities, such as classism, racism, and sexism.

Survival

In addition to understanding the needs of their community, the activists explained that another motivation for their involvement in the AIDS movement is their desire to help ensure the survival of themselves and their communities. Forty-five-year-old Rue, who worked in AIDS activism for over 25 years, elaborated, "I think it's the whole thing about Black survival in the U.S. [My activism] is part of our cultural survival. [It is] a continuation of the legacy of Blacks in America, that we had to be there for each other if we were going to sustain the race." Likewise, Latrice, a 48-year-old community educator and outreach worker for a Detroit-based community organization, discussed the care she has for her community, and, as an HIV-positive woman, how she advocates for both her community and herself. She stated, "It's because that's where my heart is, and, you know, that's where my care and my heart is. To pour out my heart to the communities and to be of service and to give back. But it's just not my total self because I have to take care of myself too, so in order to take care of myself first, I can be able to take care of somebody else." Jasmine, 51-year-old founder of a New York City-based AIDS service organization working with formerly incarcerated women, explained her motivation to engage in AIDS activism work:

I think the motivation comes from the need for survival. For the need to continue to live in a manner in which we are relevant, that we are no longer invisible, that we don't have to keep quiet, that we can hold up our banner and whatever it is, and fight. And we don't have to fade into black, that we can be a vibrant piece of, part of what's going on. And that's in the movement of Black women.

In these three cases, personal and cultural survival primarily motivated mobilization. According to the women, their AIDS activism was an attempt to address one of the many social ills within Black communities, and activism became an important part of their identity. The findings appear to be consistent with the literature pertaining to motivations for community activism among Black women (Maparyan 2012; Collins 2000).

As part of their ability to survive as a community, study participants also believed that their activism was a form of community caretaking. Forty-eight-year-old Sandy, the vice president of community development for a large AIDS service organization that works to reduce rates of HIV among Blacks, noted, "Black women tend to be the ones to care for the community because we are the ones that breathe life. It's who we are. It's bred into us to provide, to take care, to nurture. Culturally, we're built into it." In her explanation, Sandy described how she nurtures her community members because it is part of her culture to do so. Both community support and survival have contributed to Black women's AIDS activism.

Womanism provides a holistic framework that considers the many factors that influence how and why Black women mobilize against AIDS within their communities. AIDS activism challenges many of the assumptions associated with intersectionality, such as the importance of identity (i.e., racial, gender, and sexuality) in activism, and, instead, highlights the significance of community in the lives of women. For the activists in this sample, race, gender, and their intersections inform their activism and their activist identities. In other words, community support is not a value or a strategy, but it is an aspect of these respondents' identities; likewise, activism is not simply a task for these women, but part of who they are. Thus, while intersectionality has been used to inform activism, unlike womanism, intersectionality does not highlight how activism is an integral part of one's identity (See the working definitions for feminism, intersectionality, and womanism in chapter 1, figure 1).

ACTIVISM AND IDENTITY

The women in our study explained how their social conditions and their need for survival were their primary motivations for mobilizing against AIDS. However, these women did not simply engage in community activism, but, rather, they emphasized how activism became an important aspect of their identity. Women discussed their identities as activists at length and focused on how their race and gender influence their identities as activists and their activism work.

Activist Identity

The activists in this study maintained that being an AIDS activist was a significant part of their identity. This appeared to be the case regardless of the specific type of activism in which they were engaged. Rose, a 42-year-old documentary filmmaker, described herself as the following, "I see myself as a documentarian, independent filmmaker, media educator, activist."

In addition, many of the women maintain that not only did they identify as activists, but others identified them as activists as well. Forty-eight-year-old Sandy, who has worked in AIDS activism for over 18 years, noted, "I would say that's how people know me; it's as an activist." Jocelyn, a 24-year veteran of AIDS activism work who lives in New York City, indicated, "the root of who I am as a human being is to have a full life, including fighting social injustice, which means being an AIDS activist. Some Black women are fighting for reproductive choices, for immigration rights, or for lifting women out of poverty or women who are survivors of domestic violence."

Those who saw their activism as being an important part of their identity also discussed how their identity as an AIDS activist fit within a larger social justice framework. Shay, a 56-year-old counselor and peer advocate for an AIDS service organization in rural South Carolina, explains,

> *Part of being an activist is being a spokesperson that speaks out and that believes in their cause and, and going back again. I think I'm more stronger after that because I care. My whole thing is that I care about people, whether it's HIV, whether it's people that is homeless, whether it's some kind of other epidemic; people hungry. I've always been that type of person that had that caring nature about myself . . . I think that's basically how I was born.*

Shay described herself as a spokesperson who "cares" and highlighted her strength as deriving from her caring nature. Shay's agency over her actions empowers her as she derives strength from her position and her caretaking abilities (Dandridge 2004; Gilkes 2001). Thus, Shay's overall concern for her community is an example of how womanism provides a strong analytical framework to examine AIDS activism among Black women.

The women in our study provided accounts of how they saw their identity in relation to their activism work. For these women, activism was a core part of their identities and they derived a sense of strength from this activist identity.

Consequently, these individuals were empowered to mobilize around multiple issues which they believed were related to AIDS, including racism, sexism, incarceration, and economic justice. They linked these various social constraints to their personal experiences and communities. And as such, this knowledge was instrumental in their identity development.

Race and Identity

Each activist stated that being a Black woman was a significant part of who they are and this identity helped to encourage their activism. To illustrate, 51-year-old Jocelyn from New York City described herself as a "Black woman, single mother, ordained nondenominational minister, and an employee in an AIDS service organization." The women in our study also described how their understanding of the oppression they experienced as Black women helped to fuel their activism efforts. Forty-two-year-old Rose explained, "when you're part of a marginalized group, to some degree, you want to empower that minority group." Similarly, 45-year-old Autumn, an executive director of a large AIDS service organization, began her community-activism work at a young age. She remembered,

> *When I was 12 years old, I sent $5 to the Free JoAnne Chesimard [also known as Assata Shakur] Fund. I sent that $5 because I was outraged that a young woman was incarcerated and could, in fact, be a victim of a rape at the hands of prison guards. And for me, it sort of defines a moment in which I recognized that the world was not fair. When I look at the world and all that is not perfect about it, I want to make it a truly more perfect union and a more perfect world, and there are many roles to that. But one of the roles is about activating change and promoting a change that's going to make a difference.*

Autumn described how passionately she felt about social justice activist Shakur's incarceration, and her resulting need to promote social change even as a child.

The respondents also described their experiences being Black women working in AIDS activism. Thirty-year-old Marva, executive director of a New York City AIDS service organization that focuses primarily on men but provides some services and support to women, stated that she felt that the clients were "disconnected" from her because she is a Black woman. Yet, Jocelyn, 51-year-old assistant director of community relations for a large AIDS service organization, explained, "I don't feel like I'm treated differently, per se, because I'm Black. I think I'm treated differently because of what I'm *saying* . . . maybe there are some people who attribute it to being a Black female." Importantly, most of the respondents said that they felt that their work was primarily viewed as positive, although sometimes, reluctantly so, Jocelyn explained,

> *There are times where I had felt like whenever I walk into a planning meeting for AIDS service organizations they would kind of roll their eyes, like "here she comes, she's going to be disruptive and make us do things we don't want to talk about or do . . ." I really have a reputation of, "You don't want to fuck with her. She is going to do her work, and it's going to be great, but don't fuck with her." I've heard these things about me. You know, firmness and harshness has its place.*

Thus, while the women were passionate about their identities as AIDS activists, they acknowledged that their racial identities affected their experiences. Nonetheless, these women were still empowered regardless of the racial and gendered stereotypes they face.

Feminism and Activism

When asked about their perspective on feminism, only about 38% of the women in the sample (N=14) identified as feminists. Thirty-three percent (N=12) of the women did not identify as feminists and the remaining women either did not answer the question or were not familiar with the definition of feminism. When asked why she identified as a feminist, 51-year-old Jasmine, the founder of a New York City AIDS service organization, said,

> *Because I understand the struggles of women as a whole, and I support those struggles. I support women's rights. I understand that a lot of the benefits that I enjoy today as a woman were as a result of the hard work of those women before me. And so, I understand the importance and the relevance of their place in my life.*

Although she originally considered herself well-versed in feminist theory and ideology, Lanetta, a 60-year-old project coordinator for an organization for LGBTQ+ people of color in Milwaukee, explained how she learned about some of the differences in feminist ideologies:

> *In the seventies, I was involved in progressive politics at school . . . And then in 1979, right after my son was born, I went to work for a feminist organization that was responsible for a lot of the women's agencies that still exist. And I embraced feminism, and I am totally comfortable calling myself a feminist. I found out a couple of years ago that I was a second-wave feminist when one of my friends and I were asked by some third-wave feminists to talk about being second-wave feminists. And we were both scratching our heads and we were like, "What are second-wave feminists?" We had to Google it and we found out*

that's the wave after the suffrage ends, which is hilarious to us. And so, yeah.
I'm totally cool with being a feminist.

Both Jasmine and Lanetta described how they supported women's rights.
Jasmine perceived women's positions as universal struggles while Lanetta
was versed in feminist theory, worked for feminist organizations, and understood herself as a feminist.

As mentioned above, a small number of activists in the sample saw themselves as feminists. Others did not wholly identify with feminism; instead,
some were unsure about their identities as feminists or outright rejected the
notion that they were feminists. Unlike Lanetta, for example, some of the
women were unsure of the definition of feminism. Eulene, a 47-year-old New
Yorker, who works in a public interest law firm, states,

> *I think I'm a feminist in that I think that women are kind of the more evolved*
> *creatures of our race and of our society, and I firmly believe that when women*
> *are good, meaning their health is good, their education is good, their economic*
> *standing is good, the whole community, the whole everything benefits when the*
> *woman is healthy. In that sense, maybe I am a feminist.*

Seeing women as "evolved creatures," Eulene personalized feminism and
saw herself within that context. Other activists, such as Jessica, a 48-year-
old case manager at a community-based organization in Detroit, were unsure
what a feminist was, and did not know whether or not they were feminists,
even though they espoused feminist ideals, such as gender equity and wom-
en's rights. Jessica explained, "I don't know; I never heard about that. I do
know that I will walk beside you; I will not walk behind you." Jessica mentions the notion of being equal but does not consider equity as an inherently
"feminist principle."

Finally, other women were certain that they did not identify themselves as
feminists. Tammy, a 37-year-old program coordinator at a community service
organization in Philadelphia, said, "I don't consider myself to be a feminist at
all, but I'm confident that I am . . . I think my liberal bend makes me just more
susceptible in those leanings. . . . If I had to, like, put a label on me, [feminist]
probably wouldn't have been one of the labels I put, but I can so very eas-
ily see people identify me as that as well." Similarly, Roxsan, a 65-year-old
educator at a Dallas AIDS service organization, said, "No, I recognize that
women and marginalized individuals are so heavily and negatively impacted
by HIV and a social and economic condition that make it such that they are
so negatively impacted, that I work in that area, but that's about it. But I don't
think I'm a feminist at all."

Many of the women in our study were reluctant to identify as feminists. As White feminism overlooked the needs of Black women (Davis 1981) and framed issues around White middle-class women (Davis 1981; hooks 1981). Black women developed their own epistemology (Collins 2000) and political movements (Taylor 2016) that centered the needs of their communities. Epistemologies, such as womanism (Walker 1994), Black feminism (Collins 2000; hooks 1981), and intersectionality (Crenshaw 2018; Collins 2000) center Black women's experiences as a reaction against feminism. Gender oppression is not the primary form of oppression Black women experience. In line with Black feminist and intersectional literature (Crenshaw 2018), it appeared that for many of the women, being a Black woman and an activist were more important to their identities as activists than their gender identity alone.

As intersectionality dictates, identities beyond gender or race help inform activism among women of color (Chun et al. 2013; Collins 2000). Although race and gender are important identities for these women, their race and gender brought up important cultural expectations and experiences that influenced their activism. Our findings indicate that the women's identities as activists, their identity as Black women, their spirituality, and their desire for community support informed their activism. These findings are consistent with work on Black women and community activism (Maparyan 2012; Gilkes 2001). These activists understood that AIDS and other factors, such as poor education, crime, poverty, violence, and unemployment, affect Black communities. These activists also believed that their activism was a form of community caretaking, which was a natural role for women, especially Black women. Our respondents discussed how their various intersecting identities (as activists, women, and Black women) influence their activism, and their perceptions of identity and social justice. As expected, a majority of the women believed that being an activist and fighting for social justice was part of their identity.

Black feminism does mention that activism is a key component of Black women's experiences; however, our findings note that activism is not simply *what* Black women do, but rather, this activism helps define *who they are.* Collins (2002) and other Black feminists (Davis 1981; Lorde 1984a) lay the theoretical groundwork that explains the nuances behind Black women's mobilization efforts to address social ills, and that literature includes Black social movements, such as Black Lives Matter (Taylor 2016). For example, when describing Black women's activism, Collins (2002, 203) asserts,

> *Domination encompasses structural, disciplinary, hegemonic, and interpersonal domains of power. . . . These domains constitute specific sites where oppressions of race, class, gender, sexuality, and nation mutually construct one another.*

> *Understanding the complexity of Black women's activism requires understand-*
> *ing not only the need to address more than one form of oppression, but the*
> *significance of how singular and multiple forms of oppression are organized.*

Here, Collins asserts that Black women's social positions affect why they organize. To make this theoretical point concrete, Collins (2002, 204) interprets Bonnie's Thornton Dill's work on Black women labor activists by noting: "The vast majority of Black women domestic workers [in Dill's study] neither organized for better working conditions nor confronted their employers by demanding better pay—actions representing the struggle for institutional transformation—because they needed their jobs. Ensuring their families' survival came first . . ." Referencing a specific account of a Black woman domestic worker in Dill's data set, Collins explains how a Black woman worker organized against unfair working conditions: "Yet even though her [the domestic worker's] actions were constrained by the need to ensure her family's economic survival, she did challenge the rules that governed her work. Her participation in a Black female sphere of influence gave her different tools to resist, and she stimulated institutional transformation by undermining the rules governing her work" (206). Even though Collins draws from a conceptual framework that centers Black women's duties to their families (Collins 2002, 206), it was the *position* of being a Black woman (i.e., that takes care of her family) that lead to the resistance. Therefore, the *behavior* (i.e., activism) was driven by the social position rather than the individual's sense of self. For Collins, Black women share a structurally marginalized status, and they engage in activism. In contrast, the women in our study described their activism as not just centered around their own position; it was because they were structurally marginalized and cared about the people they were trying to help (i.e., other structurally oppressed community members). Thus, from this perspective, Black women engage in activism because they occupy a marginalized position comprised of intersecting structurally marginalized identities. This is, indeed, very different than saying that Black women base their identities on activism. The women in our study described that their very sense of self is shaped within the purview of activism, especially because survival, community care, and culture shape Black women's experiences.

As previously explained, the women in our study understood how the matrix of oppression (Collins 2002) disproportionately impacted their lives. Denise McLane-Davison's (2016) work examines Black women's leadership in AIDS advocacy and suggests that racial and gender identity, inclusivity, and notions of mothering influence their advocacy work. Using a Black feminist framework, McLane-Davison (2016) emphasizes how social identity (e.g., race, gender, and their intersections) impacts the experiences of

Black women. While the women in our study noted the importance of their identities as Black women, they explained that their identity *as* an activist as well as their notions of community support greatly influenced their activism and their sense of self. Even in AIDS activism literature, Black feminist and intersectional literature underemphasizes these factors. As the idea of intersectionality has its roots in the work and research of Black women, and is based on their lives and experiences, one would surmise that intersectional frameworks would apply to the experiences of the activists in this sample. Nevertheless, intersectionality appears to overlook the various nuances and complexities of their identities.

Even some womanist literature that examines social movement formation, including the Black Lives Matter movement (Richardson 2019), misses this distinction. For example, Richardson (2019) describes how "empowerment," a central womanist tenet, is a mode of communication within the Black Lives Matter movement but did not describe that this empowerment is central to Black women's *identities* as activists. Thus, the women in our study describe that their very sense of self is being a Black woman *and* an activist, and this then breaks with Black feminist, intersectional, and even some womanist literature.

CONCLUSION

The activists in our study discussed the importance of their race and gender in detail, and they emphasized how race and gender encouraged their activism. In lieu of race and gender, the respondents described their activist identity and their communities as central to their experiences. In addition, study participants spoke at length concerning how their activism was, in part, designed to benefit their communities. Not surprisingly, a majority of the activists believe that being an activist and fighting for social justice are parts of their identity.

It was notable, however, that a number of women did not identify as feminists. Black feminist scholars, such as Patricia Hill Collins (2000) and bell hooks (1981) argue that feminism overlooks the experiences and perceptions of women of color, and, unlike their White feminist counterparts, these women do not experience gender as their primary form of oppression. This appeared to be the case among several women in our sample. Womanism helps us to better understand the important role that community and activism have on the identities of the women in our study and can better explain the ways in which Black women mobilize to form more contemporary movements, such as Black Lives Matter. With womanism, we find that race, class, and gender oppression provide women of color with a unique worldview that also helps to inform not only their life experiences, but also their social justice activities. As a result, womanism more clearly helps us to ascertain how the Black women in our study understand their own identities as Black women and as activists compared to other theoretical frameworks.

Chapter Three

Religion and Spirituality in AIDS Activism

In the previous chapter, we examined how the women in our study negotiated their race, gender, and activism work. These activists also negotiated understandings of feminism with their racialized identities and emphasized group survival over notions of gender oppression. We find that womanism aptly encapsulates how Black women define themselves as activists because these activists draw upon culturally specific notions of their identities to empower themselves and their communities. Another key aspect of womanism is its emphasis on spirituality. While Black women draw on culturally specific values to create identities and social movements, such as being the caretakers of their communities, Black women have spiritual belief systems that affect both identity creation and social mobilization. This chapter examines religion and spirituality and how it influences the lives and activism of the women in our study and the role Black religious communities play in their activism efforts.

RELIGION AND SPIRITUALITY IN BLACK COMMUNITIES

Studies suggest that religion and spirituality are paramount in the lives of Black Americans, and, in particular, Black women, who report the highest rates of religiosity in the nation (Washington Post 2012; Brown and Brown 2003). Religion and spiritualty have not only eased many of the social and emotional burdens that many Black women endure as a result of discrimination and poverty, but religion and spirituality have also historically served as a motivating force for social change and community activism (Brown and Brown 2003; Frederick 2003).

A study conducted by *The Washington Post* (2012) and Kaiser Family Foundation found that "74% of [B]lack women and 70% of [B]lack men believe 'that living a religious life' is 'very important' compared to 57% of [W]hite women and 43% of [W]hite men." Furthermore, "87% of [B]lack women and 79% of [B]lack men believe that 'religion or faith in God' plays a very important role 'in helping [respondents] get through tough times' compared to 66% of [W]hite women and 51% of [W]hite men" (*Washington Post* 2012). This study also found that 84% of Black adults considered themselves to be religious, 77% reported that the church was still very important, 71% attended church at least once a month, and nearly 70% were members of a church (*Washington Post* 2012). In fact, this survey found that Black women had the highest rates of life satisfaction, with 51% reporting being very satisfied with their lives, as compared to 46% among Black men, 50% among White women, and 48% among White men (*Washington Post* 2012).

Research finds that religion and spirituality help provide a positive outlook and overall well-being (Wilson 2000). For instance, one study indicates that Blacks who attend church regularly, defined as 2–3 times a month, are healthier than Blacks who do not attend church regularly (Wilson 2000). Worshipping in a community provides social support and encourages community involvement. Black religious traditions often emphasize notions of social justice and equity for the oppressed and downtrodden (Lincoln and Mamiya 1990). In examining coping mechanisms, research finds that among professional Black women, spirituality (e.g., prayer or mediation) is often used to help deal with life's challenges (Bacchus and Holley 2005). Additionally, research finds that some HIV-positive Black women report higher levels of psychological well-being when they report higher levels of spirituality (Braxton et al. 2007). However, the stigmas associated with AIDS have been a challenge for many religious institutions within Black communities, and in particular, the Black Church.

A majority of Blacks in the United States consider themselves to be a member of one of the seven traditional denominations that are collectively known as the "Black Church" (Lincoln and Mamiya 1990). Black churches are typically characterized by their jubilant services that often encourage worship through music, song, and dance (Lincoln and Mamiya 1990). Black churches are also known for promoting liberation theology—an interpretation of Christian beliefs that emphasizes freedom, acceptance, and social justice (Cone 1996). These Black churches have helped to cultivate a culture of activism within Black communities, and, in particular, among Black women (Douglas 2018; Gilkes 2001).

Black Church culture and the emphasis on spirituality found within Black communities have provided many Black women with the encouragement and strength to seek out change to help improve their communities and fight for those in need (Gilkes 2001). Nonetheless, although AIDS is one of the leading causes of death within Black communities, many of the activists in our study have found that religious institutions impede AIDS activism work. HIV is transmitted through bodily fluids and through perceived stigmatized activities (e.g., IV drug use and unsafe sex), and Black churches were perceived to have shied away from acknowledging AIDS' negative impact on Black communities (Cohen 1999). Consequently, in order to help reduce HIV and AIDS stigma, activists have increasingly targeted Black churches to promote education and awareness (Harris 2010). Prior to their activism work, most of the women in our study were deeply involved in religious activism and were even raised in religious homes. However, their activism work has caused tensions between how they view and experience their religious identities and their spirituality.

Religion, Spirituality, and Activism

Both religion and spirituality deeply affect the lives of the activists in our study. The women in our study were raised in a religious home and identified themselves as spiritual. However, while they noted that both religion and spirituality affected their lives in different ways, they drew clear distinctions between the role that religion and spirituality play in their lives and activism work.

Family Upbringing

All of the women interviewed grew up in a home with religious and/or spiritual beliefs. For example, Tammy, a 37-year-old program coordinator in Philadelphia who has worked in AIDS activism for over 19 years, said, "I am a preacher's child and a granddaughter of a preacher. The niece of, like, 15 preachers." Isabella, a 41-year-old women's program coordinator in Los Angeles, explained that her upbringing "wasn't religious, it was more spiritual, I was raised in church, but not, like, *in church*. You know what I mean?" Sandy, a 45-year-old vice president for communication for a New York City AIDS service organization explained, "We do practice, and it is a practice. It's more around the philosophy. I think my parents are still religious. It wasn't necessarily about the Bible, but more about understanding the principles and how you begin to internalize one so you can think of it as a way to guide your life and how you interact and interface with others." Other women, such as 66-year-old Ena, who founded a nonprofit for sex workers, were not raised practicing mainstream Christianity. Ena explains, "[B]eing a Jehovah Witness, I didn't like it, put it that way [laughs]. My mother and father were Jehovah Witness. When I was, like, nine and 10, I didn't go to church. They didn't go to church. But I think, when I was about 10, my daddy started to go to the Jehovah Witness. But I never liked it. I never liked it."

Even for women like Ena, who were raised in families where regular church attendance was not enforced, they were still raised in what they felt were deeply religious homes. This religiosity had a deep impact on not only their upbringing, but their identity formation and understandings of their own spiritualty.

Distinctions between Religiosity and Spirituality

With the exception of one activist, most of the respondents identified themselves as either spiritual or religious, with varying degrees of church attendance. However, one woman, Lanetta, a 60-year-old health project coordinator from Milwaukee, described herself as a "humanist" and "not particularly religious" despite being raised in what she referred to as a spiritual family.

Even though religion and religious beliefs clearly affected these women's lives, most did not identify as religious. Twenty-one out of the 36 women interviewed in our study identified as spiritual instead of religious. Fifty-year-old Oakland-based peer advocate Dorothy maintained that she was not religious: "I feel like God knows my heart. I feel like God knows my heart so I don't feel like I need to go into a building to communicate. I just don't, you know? I just don't." In fact, a number of the women described church as being just a "building." Fifty-eight-year-old Orangeburg, South Carolina-based program coordinator Brianna, who has worked in AIDS activism for 18 years, explained, "Well, the church is a building. I'm about spirituality and God is the head of my life. I do go to a church, but the pastor is not the king of my life because he's just a man. A lot of times, rules and regulations that people have in the church, I may not follow them because I feel as my conviction comes from the man up above." Also identifying as a spiritual person and not religious, and founder of a New York City AIDS service organization targeting women and children, 51-year-old Jasmine articulated her understanding of the role of both the church and the pastor in her life:

> I'm a very spiritual person. I believe in my higher power. I understand the role
> of church or organized religion in my community, but I don't—and I have to be
> really honest—I don't ascribe to that . . . I understand that the man standing in
> the pulpit is just a man and he is the messenger bringing the word of God and
> nothing more. That I'm able to understand, the church is not that building. The
> church is where my heart is, and I bring church with me whereever I go. So,
> while it plays a significant role [in my life], it doesn't.

Although these women indicated that they were not religious, like Jasmine, they believed in a higher power. Alyssa, an AIDS service worker from New York City, stated: "I was raised Catholic, but I'm not religious. I'm not in church every Sunday or anything like that, but I would consider myself to be a highly spiritual person, you know that there is something much bigger than all of us." Some of these women indicated that their spirituality extends beyond just their belief in God. Rue, a 45-year-old unemployed activist from Boston, described herself as, "Spiritual, not Christian. I like gospel music and I play it often but I'm very uncomfortable with the dogma of Christianity. I have been exposed to other religions and I guess I do take bits and pieces of things that make sense to me and to some extent help sustain me or give me a different way about thinking about my challenges." Glenda, a New York City-based community educator, stated, "I have a lot of spiritual symbols at home. I wear a crucifix because I do believe in that. I feel it. I know it's there. I know I have ancestors; I know they watch over me." In these cases, the activists made clear distinctions between religion and spirituality, emphasizing the importance of their spiritual identities in the process.

In addition to discussing the impact that religion and spirituality have had on their lives and upbringing, the women also discussed religious institutions within Black communities, and, in particular, the Black Church, and how these institutions—by delaying their response to HIV in Black communities—inadvertently helped fuel rates of HIV in these communities. They also discussed how Black churches and other religious institutions can be used to help combat AIDS within Black communities.

The Black Church

As noted above, religion and spirituality heavily influenced the lives of these activists. Most of these activists grew up in an environment that extolled religiosity. While the women emphasized their spirituality, all respondents had been involved with formal religious institutions, and, in particular, the Black Church, which affected how they understood religion, spirituality, and AIDS discourse. In their discussion of the Black Church, these women either critiqued the Black Church and discussed the negative impact it had on their activism work or provided a series of suggestions to get churches involved in AIDS education and community advocacy.

Challenges

The women in our study often distinguished between being religious and spiritual because of the oppressive role they felt that religion, and, in particular, the Black Church, has on their AIDS activism efforts and community outreach. Many of these women felt that the Black Church created barriers that prevent AIDS education and affected how the respondents perceived the Church. Rue stated, "I actually think Christianity has been a big road block for us as a community, I think . . . as a Black community, I believe it has been a major fucking road block." Jocelyn, a New York City AIDS community educator in her fifties, stated, "I hear that people say that AIDS is God's punishment, and my commitment is that I will continue to try to do this work until people will stop saying that AIDS is God's punishment because that is so disgusting, and so tragic, so horrendous, that it speaks to the holocaust that the epidemic is." The respondents also discussed how religion hinders their individual AIDS activism efforts. New York City AIDS activist Alyssa explained, "I understand that certain practices are because of certain religious beliefs and if you're talking to somebody about condom use and they are like, 'Well, in my religion we don't use condoms,' that's a real challenge to get through because you don't want to tell the person, 'Well, don't practice your religion.' But you also want them to understand the importance of using a condom or eliminating some of those sex partners or something like that." Jocelyn, a New York City activist who has worked in AIDS activism for over 26 years, maintains that part of her challenge is working with religious organizations:

A lot of the clergy do not want to do this work. [They] do not want to talk about sex. They do not want to talk about substance abuse. They do not want to talk about the link of sex and religion, they just don't. It's really like trying to go into a cult oftentimes and you are either trying to take the clergy down or trying to "un-brainwash" the people who go to the faith community. It's just horrible but such necessary work. Some of the Black churches have been telling the same lies to their congregations for 20 years, 25 years, 30 years, then along came an AIDS activist and you know, you can't keep saying this, that homosexuality is bad. It's just you can't. It's a public health emergency. I am sorry, you can't do it. You're helping to raise the infection honey, sorry.

Jessica, a 48-year-old case manager from Detroit who has worked in AIDS activism for nine years, complained, "Half of the churches don't even want to talk about HIV and AIDS and when they do . . . [they] make it seem like it's a bad thing."

The activists critiqued the Black Church's negative treatment and ostracism of HIV-positive individuals. Marva described the experiences a number of her clients have with the Black Church:

A lot of times when you talk to the clients they will tell you they're still shunned from the Church. That will be one of the first topics they [discuss] talking to them. And if they grow up in the Church, especially, a lot of Blacks who were raised in the South, [Church] was part of everyday. . . . It contributes to the shame that they already feel. A lot of the time when you think of Black Church, especially within our communities, you think of a place for families. . . . So, if the Black Church can embrace individuals in these communities, can you imagine how much hope they can actually instill into these individuals so they can make it another day?

For many of the women, religion poses a challenge when working in Black AIDS organizations. While laughing, Boston-based activist, Rue, explained, "One of the challenges I really do have in working within Black organizations is they would begin every meeting with a prayer. I did everything I could to avoid it. If I could get there and put my pen and pencil down so they know I was there and then as people would come in, I'd sneak out and go stand in the bathroom for like five minutes or something until that part would be over."

Interestingly, although many of the activists critiqued Black churches, many of them were active in these religious institutions, such as was the case with Roxsan, the 65-year-old Dallas-based peer educator, who is actively involved in "six different ministries" at her church. Additionally, these women also are aware of the important role that the Black Church plays in the lives of Blacks and their communities. Although frustrated, many women displayed an understanding of the challenges that Black churches have in addressing HIV. In discussing the challenges the Church faces, while also highlighting the specific role of Black women in the Church, Glenda, from New York City, explained,

> *I think they're trying. I think that some churches are doing very well, and there are just some churches who are doing miserably, and those in the middle who are starting their ministries or had their health ministries or their service to the people. I just think that, I want to be honest with you, the Church is tired too! Think, who runs the Church? Black women! They tired! I see them; they're tired! They're tired. They got a lot on their shoulders, they need a break too! I think they're trying to do the best that they can, and it's not that I don't want to say anything bad about them. I honestly really feel as if they are giving all that they can give and that there is not enough people coming back up through the ranks for a whole lot of reasons. You know?*

These critiques of the Black Church and the activists' work (or lack thereof) with Black churches appeared to impact the religious and/or spiritual identities of the participants in this study. As noted by a number of activists, the Black Church's response to the AIDS epidemic made them question how religious discourse impacts those most in need. Although the women believed in a higher power and recognized how it affected their lives, a vast majority identified as spiritual. They also emphasized the importance between the two. As the activists noted, religious institutions overall (Harris 2010), including the Black Church, were not immediately supportive of those groups stereotyped as being infected with HIV. Overt homophobia (Kornegay 2004), and stigmas surrounding homosexuality, promiscuity, and drug use prevented most, but not all, Black Church leaders and congregants from immediately addressing AIDS in Black communities (Harris 2010). Nonetheless, it is important to note that spirituality and the belief in a higher power were still central to the respondents' activism.

Regardless of the Black Church's emphasis on social justice (Cone 1996), one of the reasons why many of the women in our study distinguished their spirituality from institutionalized religion was because of the perpetual homophobia and sexism they witnessed in religious institutions. Nonetheless, their spirituality still helped motivate them to engage in AIDS activism work and engage with religious institutions in these efforts. Potentially, as argued in the previous chapter, this could be because the women in our study emphasized community care (Walker-Barnes 2014), their culture, and their identities as Black women; therefore, the needs of their community superseded their own experiences with religion.

WOMANISM AND SPIRITUALITY

As discussed, religion and spirituality heavily impacted the lives of the women in our study. Given their histories, these women noted that oppressive structures, such as sexism and homophobia, limited their participation in the Black Church, while still maintaining that the Black Church was a strong influence in their lives and upbringing. Black churches may have traditionally avoided discussions of AIDS, but they have cultivated a culture of activism among Black women (Gilkes 2001). Black Church culture and the emphasis on spirituality found within Black communities have provided many Black women with the encouragement and strength to seek out change to help improve their communities (Gilkes 2001). Findings indicated that both religion and spirituality impacted their activism; however, respondents noted that religion hinders their AIDS activism while their spirituality provides them with strength and encouragement.

Separate from religion, spirituality emphasizes the belief not necessarily in a higher power, but in an overarching interconnectedness between living beings. Oftentimes, spirituality is used as a means of self-empowerment. According to Maparyan (2012), there are three important principles of spiritual activism: "(1) the Innate Divinity of humans and creation; (2) the existence and lawfulness of the invisible realm; and (3) humans as energy transformers who can 'perform' miracles by learning and applying metaphysical laws that are encapsulated within the world's mystical and esoteric wisdom traditions" (141). All of the women, including the women who did not identify as religious or spiritual, believed in this "higher power." Additionally, most respondents also believed in their ability to "transform" the social world and understood this ability to be a divine gift. Although research already notes how religion and spirituality have hampered AIDS activism efforts and promoted AIDS stigma (Herek and Capitanio 1999; Fullilove et al. 1990), womanism emphasizes religion and spirituality's role in AIDS activism. Often portrayed as a challenge in AIDS activism efforts, religion and spirituality can also motivate Black women to engage in social change. For instance, all but one of these women noted that a "higher power" motivated their activism.

A key component of womanism is its acknowledgement of the importance of spirituality in the lives of women of color and its provision of a deeper theoretical lens through which to examine Black women's activism and spirituality: "Womanism openly acknowledges a spiritual/transcendental realm with which human life, living kind, and the material world are all intertwined. . . . [S]piritual intercession and consideration of the transcendental or metaphysical dimension of life enhance and even undergird political action" (Phillips 2006). In womanism, this blend of spirituality and activism, where activists put their "spirituality to work for positive social and ecological change" (Phillips 2006) is referred to as "spiritual activism" (Maparyan 2012). Although womanism provides a theoretical framework to examine activism, it has been underutilized in empirical studies that examine social activism among Black women.

Spirituality and Womanism

Spirituality is central to womanist thought and has an extensive range of literature that focuses on theology (Baker-Fletcher 2014) in social movements (Buhuro 2018). In terms of its intersections, womanist spirituality has been examined in relation to Black Catholicism (Hayes 2016). Spirituality has also been examined within the context of Black women, their bonds with one another (Williams 2013), and their roles as community caretakers and burden-bearers (Walker-Barnes 2014; Gilkes 2001). Womanist spirituality has also been applied in multiple efforts, including connecting with the environment (Harris 2017), dismantling oppressive structures, such as racism and police brutality, and advocating for transformative justice politics (Buhuro 2018; Kaba 2021). Womanist spirituality has also highlighted queer experiences (Lightsey 2015) and AIDS (Anderson 2016). In her work, rather than focusing on activists, Anderson's (2016) work examined issues of sexism and homophobia within Black churches and provided a womanist interpretation of the Bible and how it applies to AIDS.

Spiritual Activism

It is key to note that all of the women in our study emphasized that their spiritualty or "humanism," as Lanetta maintained earlier, greatly informed their AIDS activism work. As New York City-based AIDS community educator Glenda explained, she expressed her spirituality through her activism, "My spirituality, my religion is my work. I'm here to serve. That's what Jesus said, serve your fellow man." Forty-seven-year-old Eulene, who works for a public interest law firm in New York City, maintained, "It's all about service. It's all about I'm doing my purpose that God has for me." For some, like Eulene, their activism served a God-given *purpose.* Many of the women also believed that they received a special "calling" to do AIDS activism work. Forty-one-year-old Los Angeles-based women's program coordinator Isabella maintained, "Yeah, I definitely know that God has called me to do this. I say that because [of] the impact that I have had on people's lives and the doors I have opened and opportunities I have been given." Dana, a 59-year-old Philadelphia-based AIDS and women's rights activist, noted that "definitely, there's a divine presence in the work that I do. I couldn't do this without being grounded in a spiritual belief . . . I have so much to give and I don't even know where it came from, but I know that I can't keep it because it's too wonderful, you know? It's called hope."

Also, for a number of these women, their spiritual beliefs grounded their work and provided them with a great deal of strength and, as New York City-based AIDS activist Alyssa described, "It helps me to be patient. . . . I think it helps [me] with people in general. To help understand people in general." Likewise, Grace, a case manager from New Orleans, stated that not only was her spirituality the "driving force" behind her activism, but it also provided her with the ability to "meet people where they are. I don't let my opinions infringe upon anybody's rights." Grace continued, "It's kind of hard to explain spirituality because people think it's like this New Age thing, and it really isn't. I respect every living thing on Earth, from a flea to a blue whale. I respect it. And having said that, that's why I'm effective at what I do, because I do respect all different things."

The women in our study directly addressed how spirituality impacted their lives. In line with the literature (Maparyan 2012), the women reported that a higher power influenced their activism. While the women in our study briefly mentioned aspects of scripture (Baker-Fletcher 2014), they also demonstrated how the "calling" they received from a "higher power" gave them purpose and influenced their activism (Marparyan 2012), and, indeed, enabled them to mobilize for their communities. Likewise, some of the women mentioned their connection with the earth and all living things (Harris 2017; Phillips 2006).

The women in this study describe in detail how their spirituality motivated them to mobilize. While they described their spirituality and its effect on their activism, the women did not specifically link their belief in God or a higher power with countering specific structures of racism (Buhuro 2018; Kaba 2021). In this data set, the women discussed racism (Buhuro 2018; Kaba 2021) and described how their identities were largely shaped by their racial identities, but not in the context of a spiritual endeavor or liberation theology (Cone 1996). Instead, they marshaled their spirituality as part of community care (Walker 1994), with the goal of dismantling all oppressive structures. Furthermore, the women in our study did not explicitly link their spirituality to their experiences as Black women (Williams 2013), but, rather connected it to their culture, communities, and families (Gilkes 2001).

CONCLUSION

Both religion and spirituality impacted the respondents' community outreach; however, respondents clearly distinguished between religion and spirituality. They also noted that religion hampers their AIDS activism work while their spirituality provides them with strength and encouragement to endure in their community activism efforts. Importantly, findings also highlight the tensions between claiming religious versus spiritual identities among the women.

Although research already notes how religion and spirituality have hampered AIDS activism efforts in and out of Black communities (Harris 2010) and have promoted AIDS stigma (Herek and Capitanio 1999; Fullilove et al. 1990), womanism enables us to see the influences that religion and spirituality have on the AIDS activism of the women in our study. Furthermore, other scholarship has applied womanism in terms of Biblical interpretation (Anderson 2016) and applied this to AIDS. In comparison, our study focuses on the experiences of the women in our study and their activism efforts. Compared to intersectionality, a womanist framework underscores how religion and spirituality impact how Black women shape their identities and mobilize against AIDS. Importantly, the response that many religious institutions have had toward HIV highlights the tensions between religion and spirituality among these women; it is clear that the belief in a higher power serves as the motivating force and encourages AIDS activism. Nonetheless, the women appear to find the institutional aspects of the religion to be somewhat oppressive to their work.

Chapter Four

Emotions

Love, Anger, and Solidarity

Audre Lorde (1984a) forcefully spoke out about the power of emotions. She believed that they help people see different possibilities and help fuel community change. Research on emotions and affect explain how emotions and feelings are important facilitators of activism. A key factor that motivated the advocacy work of the women in our study was simply the feelings they had for their loved ones and their communities. In this chapter, we will examine the role emotions play in fueling community activism and advocacy and how emotions impact the work of the women in our study and help drive their desire for social change.

EMOTIONS AND ACTIVISM

Social scientists have long examined the role of emotions and the impact they have on social interactions, while also contending that the number of emotions that people exhibit vary—some suggest there are three emotions while others argue that there are as many as 11 emotions (Plutchik 2003). Theories of primary emotions typically focus on anger, love, fear, sadness, and happiness (Plutchik 2003). Sociologist Peggy Thoits (1989) notes that definitions of emotions tend to refer to a series of components consisting of the following: (a) "appraisals . . . stimulus or context," (b) "changes in . . . bodily sensations," (c) "the "display of expressive gestures," and (d) "a cultural label applied to . . . one or more of the first three components" (318). Thoits (1989) explains the differences between emotions and affects:

> *Emotions can be distinguished from feelings, affects, moods, and sentiments. The first two are less specific terms, the latter two, more specific. The term,*

45

"feelings," includes the experience of physical drive states (e.g., hunger, pain, fatigue) as well as emotional states. Affects refer to positive and negative evaluations (liking/disliking) of an object, behavior, or idea; affects also have intensity and activity dimensions. Thus, emotions can be viewed as culturally delineated types of feelings or affects. (1989, 318)

As such, emotions involve physiological responses to the external stimuli and cultural interpretation.

Emotions and Women

In sociology, emotions have been viewed from a variety of perspectives. For example, symbolic interactionists argue that cues, which vary based on situation, determine one's emotions (Schachter and Singer 1962). Similarly, social constructionists argue that social and cultural forces construct how we understand, experience, and feel emotions (Armon-Jones 1986). According to Arlie Russell Hochschild (1979), women are often expected to suppress their own emotions and induce context-dependent emotional displays in an effort to manage others' emotions. Calling this "emotion work," Hochschild (1979) argues that this emotional labor is added labor that goes into caring for and managing the emotions of others and is most often assigned to women. Often, this labor is commodified (Hochschild 1979; 2010). Importantly, Hochschild (1979) also maintains that much of the emotion and the emotion work women experience is based on cultural expectations and norms. Hochschild does not explicitly address race in this analysis and how race and gender impact emotional responses (Hochschild 1979). Shields et al. (2006) argue that "a number of beliefs about gender difference are grounded in beliefs about the emotional nature of each sex, particularly the way in which emotionality marks female/feminine as different from male/masculine" (63). As such, women are expected to be both more emotional and engage in more emotional labor. Not only can emotions be governed by societal expectations and norms (Plutchik 2003), they can serve as important motivators for social justice and community activism (Gould 2009).

Social movement scholars examine the emotions that drive the activism work that leads to social movements and societal change (Goodwin and Jasper 2006; Hoggett 2015). Displays of frenzied emotion inspired early social movement theorists to categorize the behavior of many activists as irrational (Goodwin and Jasper 2006; Jenkins 1983). In their attempt to shift social movement theory away from framings of irrational behavior as motivation for collective behavior, theorists argued that this behavior was, instead, rational (Goodwin and Jasper 2006). Consequently, social movement scholarship has traditionally overlooked the role that emotions have played in motivating activism and protest over the past few decades (Goodwin and Jasper 2006).

Resource mobilization theory, a key social movement framework, emerged to counter the belief in framings of irrationality found in collective behavior theory (Jenkins 1983; Tilly 2017). Research mobilization theory argues that activists use emotions to help frame social issues and problems in ways that resonate with the target audience and other sympathizers and activists. By reframing emotions as rational, social movement scholars argued that these theorists overlooked the impact that emotions play in motivating activism work. As such, this perspective argues that emotions are not irrational, but, rather, are rational and instrumental in achieving movement goals. In fact, scholars argued that inducing an emotional response to an issue was a factor used by social movement actors to shape an event or issue to fit one's world-view and one's perceptions of justice or injustice (Snow and Benford 1992). These actors framed social movements to elicit further support and better understandings of the social injustices motivating their behavior. For example, while Gamson (1992) argued that injustice itself is a frame, these frames are contingent upon "the righteous anger that puts fire in the belly and iron in the soul" (32). Thus, individuals do not simply act on emotions out of irrationality, but, rather, deploy emotions instrumentally while engaging in activism.

Black Women's Emotions and Activism

Although Black women have always been deeply engaged in social justice work (Froyum 2010), research overlooks the influence of emotions and feelings on Black women's activism. Much of the emotion women experience is based on cultural expectations and norms (Hochschild 1979). Calling this "emotion work," Hochschild (1979) argues that this emotional labor is added labor that goes into caring for and managing the emotions of others and is most often assigned to women. Often, this labor is commodified (2010). Research extends this notion to study the additional emotional labor that Black women perform (Durr and Wingfield 2011). Although research examines how Black women care for the emotions of others, research overlooks their own emotions.

Culture helps us understand "what constitutes an emotion" (Peterson 2006, 115). Additionally, culture contributes to how individuals identify and express emotions (Rosenberg 1990; 1991). Activist and Black feminist scholar Audre Lorde (1984a, 127) explained that emotions, anger in particular, can be used in a positive way to help fuel social change. She writes:

Every woman has a well-stocked arsenal of anger potentially useful against those oppressions, personal and institutional, which brought that anger into

being. Focused with precision it can become a powerful source of energy serv-
ing progress and change. And when I speak of change, I do not mean a simple
switch of positions or a temporary lessening of tensions, nor the ability to smile
or feel good. I am speaking of a basic and radical alteration in those assump-
tions underlining our lives.

Other Black women scholars and activists (Davis 1981; Wells 2002) have
recognized Black women's gender, racial, class, and sexual oppression as
the root of the "anger" that Black women experience, and this helps influence their activism. In social justice movements, Black women mobilized
against sexism in Black activist organizations and racism in feminist organizations (Weisenfeld 1997; White 1999). Additionally, women's activism
in the civil rights movement was documented (Olson 2001) just as was
the sexism they experienced at the hands of Black men in this movement
(Dyson 2008). Nonetheless, from the abolitionist movement to the Black
Lives Matter movement, Black women have been either at the forefront
or have been active members of every social justice movement targeting
women and Blacks in America. Social justice organizations and movements
started by Black women include National Coalition of 100 Black Women,
National Council of Negro Women, National Welfare Rights Organization,
Brotherhood of Sleeping Car Porters, National Congress of Black Women,
Inc., National Association of Colored Women's Clubs, and National Black
Feminist Organization.

Anger also played a key role in Black women's involvement in health
activism as Black women were particularly active in health and reproductive
rights movements (Smith 1995). Having faced racism and sexism in health
reform movements, in 1983, a group of Black women medical professionals,
health care workers, researchers, and laypersons created the National Black
Women's Health Project (Morgen 2002). This organization was one in a long
line of organizations created by Black women to address health inequities
within their communities and where they could serve in leadership positions
(Hammonds 1995; Smith 1995). Community health workers, health care
providers, midwives, and doulas provided reproductive health information to
Black women to counter "the racist ideology of the mainstream, White-led
birth control movement" (Morgen 2002, 51).

Emotion theorist Deborah Gould (2009) argued that emotions and feelings
are a principal part of any social movement, as they often heavily influence
the behaviors and responses of social justice advocates (Gould 2009). She
found that the shame that those infected with HIV were made to feel about
themselves, their sexuality, and their identity helped to fuel, "outrageous, in-
your-face, sexy, and angry activism" (Gould 2009, 191). This anger helped
to inspire a sense of community and solidarity, or what she referred to "as af-

finities and reciprocities across difference" (329). It was this very difference, Gould writes, that caused the ultimate "fracturing" of the AIDS ACT UP movement and led to its decline (Gould 2009). Gould (2009) and Hochschild (1983) emphasize the importance that identity and culture play in influencing the emotions that encourage people to mobilize to enact social change. However, as previously noted, few studies examine the ways in which emotion motivates activism and community engagement among women of color, and, in particular, Black women.

In addition to how anger impacts Black women's activism, many Black women feel a sense of responsibility, attachment, and love for their communities and this attachment is integral to their sense of identity (Gilkes 2001; Collins 2000). As discussed in the first two chapters, Black women have been charged as community caretakers and have frequently fought for the well-being of their children, families, loved ones, and communities. Collins (2000) explains that this "othermothering" is an important aspect of Black culture. Gilkes (2001) argues that the importance of community care has been instilled in Black women from their youth and has become a key part of Black American culture. Black women's activism and community engagement have become cultural expectations that are necessary for community survival (Collins 2000; Gilkes 2001). As such, scholars have emphasized the support and care Black women provide their communities and their ability to quickly mobilize to address community concerns (Giddens 1996; McLane-Davidson 2016). For example, Weisenfeld (1997) argues that much of the activism and community engagement among Black women was a response to the lack of services and governmental support provided to Black communities. Consequently, Black women provided this necessary community care and support (Weisenfeld 1997). Weisenfeld (1997, 14) writes:

> *Enslaved African American women developed networks to support each other in childbirth, childrearing, and the provision of health care, in addition to assisting Black men to meet their own needs. Their free counterparts during the same period organized female benevolent societies, reading groups, antislavery societies, and religious associations to provide similar services to free Blacks.*

Feminist theory has long been interested in how emotion impacts the experiences of women. Although there has been a call to recognize the unique contributions and experiences of Black women and women of color in affect studies, or the study of emotions, the work and contribution of women of color has been under-studied and under-examined (Carrillo-Rowe and Royster 2017). Carrillo-Rowe and Royster (2017, 243) argue that "within the context of U.S. settler colonial culture, queer women of color bear the burden of affect, saturated by the colonial gaze with emotional excess: angry, hyper-sexual, depressed, dysfunctional." They argue that the emotional gaze is often from the perspective of White men, where White men determine "appropriate" and "inappropriate" displays of emotion within given situations. However, shifting the emotional gaze to Black women will help us provide an alternative view for community change. Our data analysis finds that the key emotions that drive AIDS activism and advocacy among the women in our study are feelings of love, anger, and solidarity. The following sections discuss these feelings in more detail and how they impact the lives of the women in our study.

Love

In her four-part definition and description of womanism, Alice Walker (1994) uses the word "love" 11 times. In our interviews with the women, feelings of love and compassion (or empathy) were the emotions expressed and discussed most frequently. There were a variety of different types of love and empathy described: the love they felt for themselves, for family and friends, and for community members. Over half of the women in the sample mentioned that they became involved in AIDS social justice work in an effort to obtain better services and treatment for themselves and other Black women in similar positions. Tara, a 59-year-old executive director of an AIDS service organization in Oakland, said, "Honestly, I think we're involved [in AIDS activism work] to save our own lives and our family's lives. We understand what this is doing to our community. I think Black women who do this work are women who, I think, really love and value other Black women, and see the injustice and are not willing to accept it. They are compelled to make a difference." Thirty-one-year-old Tracy, who works in AIDS outreach and advocacy in Philadelphia, explained,

I think with most AIDS activism work, if you've been infected, that's really what pushes a lot of people toward working with [AIDS]. And if you know someone who is infected, I think that is part of it. And then if you just have a concern for the overall, the people that are around you, if you, yourself, are involved in relationships and you're concerned with the men in your lives, the women in your lives, if you have little brothers, sisters, cousins, whatever, you feel that connection to teach others because you have young ones or people that you want to protect, I think that motivates people to get involved. But I think the majority of people, especially dealing with HIV and AIDS, the main thing that kind of motivates a lot of them is that they themselves have been infected, and then that pushes them to become involved.

Forty-eight-year-old Latrice, an AIDS outreach worker from Detroit, describes what motivates her, "to give back. That's the motivation, to give back. That you want to give, you want to give back, you want to give something of yourself that you never gave before, and that's, that's to love another person, to let them know that you don't have to get [HIV]." Fifty-one-year-old Jocelyn, who works in community education in New York City, explained that she became involved in AIDS activism because a former lover became infected with HIV. She noted,

> *My friends were dying. I am from the era of people dying in '81, '82 in the early years. The first love of my life when I met him, he was a bisexual, but then years later kind of crossed over to being completely gay, but you know he was the first love of my life and you know his name is Max and he died of AIDS. We had grown apart, you know, when I first dated him, I dated him in '78, '79 he was just an amazing human being. He just went on just being with men; that was sad, but some of the best people in this world died who contributed extraordinary music, art, politics, theatre. And it's just heart-wrenching some of the best lovers of life died and it's just seemed so incredible to believe, unfair and unjust that they had to die, you know? And I just don't get that and so like in any kind of disaster I was like what can I do? I have to do something.*

Whether, as Jocelyn explained, "it's about people dying that I love," or as Jessica, a 48-year-old case manager from Detroit, articulated, "Because we're finally learning how to care about ourselves and others, and we want to help," it is clear that love was at the root of their activism efforts.

The idea of caring and loving oneself was important to the women. For example, 59-year-old peer educator Shanice explained that she had to learn to love herself and see that she has value. When positing suggestions for how to promote self-love among Black women, Shanice suggests, "Number one, education. Self-awareness. Loving thyself." Shanice goes on to explain how she developed this mentality: "You know, ever since I was small, when I was in second or third grade, my father—who was born in 1913—stated, 'Number one, marriage. Gotta have a husband.' And then my father went through that, you know, 'Make sure he's light skinned and got good hair, so your kids will have light skin and good hair and be pretty.'" Even after enduring her father's sexism, colorism, and internalized racism, she understood that she was valuable and worthy of love. A notion that she works to promote to other Black women as part of her activism.

With few exceptions (Goode 1959; Hochschild 1979), sociological research on love has been understudied (Felmlee and Sprecher 2006). Sociologists argue that love is an emotion "that occurs in a relationship" (Felmlee and Sprecher 2006, 391). For example, explaining how compassion and social relations influence activism work, 31-year-old Tracy from Philadelphia explained, "If you, yourself, are involved in relationships and you're concerned with the men in your lives, the women in your lives, if you have little brothers, sisters, cousins, whatever, you feel that connection to teach others because you have young ones or others that you want to protect." Similarly, as noted above, Jocelyn described that it was her lover's HIV infection that caused her to become an activist. She said, "He was the first love of my life . . . and he died of AIDS." Jocelyn explained that her love for Max inspired her AIDS activism. Not only did the activists reference love as their primary motivation, it was also the most emphasized emotion described by Walker in her four-part definition of womanism. As Walker (1994) emphasizes, a womanist loves herself and others. She writes that a womanist "[l]oves music, Loves dance. Loves the moon. *Loves* the Spirit. Loves love and food and roundness. Loves struggle. *Loves* the Folk. Loves herself. *Regardless*" (Walker 1994, xii). Here, Walker explains that it is love for herself, love for her body, and love for her people, community, and culture that motivate womanists. And it would appear to motivate the activists in our study as well.

Anger

Throughout the interviews, the activists expressed their frustration and anger, and this was often juxtaposed against the love they felt for their communities. This anger was especially evident when asked how they initially became involved in their AIDS social justice work. Eulene, a 47-year-old activist from New York City who works in a public interest law firm, discussed how angry she was when she started her activism:

> You know, I tell people that I still am angry. I was angry from the very beginning, like I was angry from the very beginning. I was angry that people were stupid about sex. I was angry that people were saying horrible things about drug users. I've been angry. The anger has been a big catalyst. That's what keeps me doing the work.

Throughout the interviews, women discussed the anger they felt toward the government, religious leaders and congregants, and community organizations and groups. Eulene believes that activism begins with a "personal insult" and explained,

> I think it starts with the personal. It has to. Maybe not has to, but it definitely starts with some kind of personal insult that things are a certain way. . . . There were people that I had the experience working around [she then names a local community activist]. She was a well-known obstetrician, but she became an activist around a host of issues because she was primarily serving Black women in Harlem and what she kept seeing unaddressed by other health care providers and by other social services, she started speaking out about it. She ended up

becoming, you know, that's the danger too, that when we're really angry, we get written off as stringent and as, you know, kind of not able to be constructive, quote unquote. So, what motivates us, I think it's totally individual, but it's gotta have something to do, or at least in my experience, and with the people I've worked with and the women I've worked with, it's just an unwillingness to accept a kind of that's just the way it is.

The women in our study also discussed their anger at the treatment of those infected. Forty-six-year-old Grace, a medical case manager from New Orleans, said that she began her activism work in the late 1980s when she became "angry" that clinics identified AIDS patients by their first and last names and would call their names out in the clinic waiting rooms. Ena, a 66-year-old Oakland-based activist and former sex worker, became involved in AIDS activism because she was frustrated with the additional marginalization that AIDS stigma caused for sex workers. She said:

Well with HIV specifically, was the fact that first they were scapegoating sex workers, so that got me involved with it, got me kind of angry and I knew that in order to make a difference I had to show my face because a lot of the women that I was working with were not African American. And to really make a difference, I felt like African Americans needed to have a voice, and lots of people, most people, don't want to talk about sex work if they have been involved in it. And so, being that my family and my friends and other people knew what my background was and didn't have a problem with it, I felt like I really needed to be out there.

The activists also discussed their awareness of being perceived as "angry." Forty-eight-year-old Sandy from New York City discusses how the "angry Black woman" trope influences her work:

I think people think because I am a Black woman and I do this work and I'm extremely angry, that's how I'm going to approach them, the Black woman, that I'm angry. That we talk in very sort of hostile, aggressive ways. I think because of the social work of Black woman, people think automatically I'm going to have a bleeding heart or that I'm not going to be able to differentiate between right and wrong cause you know, oh, poor baby. I think as a Black woman doing this work you know you deal with sexism as it sort of comes.

Here we see how perceptions of one respondent's anger influence her activism and interactions with others.

Unlike love, there is a significant amount of scholarship on the impact that anger has on behavior and interaction. Similar to love, anger is a "social" emotion (Schieman 2006; Kemper 1987). Schieman (2006) contends that "common elicitors of anger involve actual or perceived insult, injustice,

betrayal, inequity, unfairness, goal impediments, the incompetent actions of
another and being the target of another person's verbal or physical aggres-
sion" (495). The women discussed their anger and frustration with society's
conservative approaches toward sex and sex education. For these women,
these responses prevented AIDS education information and resources from
being readily available within their communities. Importantly, the women
were aware that Black women are viewed as angry, and these views influenced their work and interactions with others.

Audre Lorde notes that it is the "fear" of Black women's anger (1984a) that
prevents an open discussion of the issues that will lead to social change. As
such, embracing fear and allowing oneself to feel angry allows one to con-
front racism and discrimination in one's life and community, and, in essence,
is a form of self-care and self-love. Lorde (1984a) states,

> *Anger expressed and translated into action in the service of our vision and our
> future is a liberating and strengthening act of clarification, for it is in the pain-
> ful process of this translation that we identify who are our allies, with whom we
> have grave differences, and who are our genuine enemies. Anger is loaded with
> information and energy.* (127)

Here, Lorde described anger as a motivating force for Black women to
pursue social change. Anger was absent from Walker's four-part definition
of womanism, but anger was heavily emphasized by Lorde as something
activists could harness to help them focus and motivate change. However,
the frustration and anger expressed by the women in our study work in tan-
dem, since, for womanists, tears are a "natural counter-balance of laughter"
(Walker 1994, xii).

Solidarity

As discussed in chapter 1, Alice Walker notes that womanists are "committed to the survival of both males and females and [desire] a world where
men and women can coexist" (Walker 1994, xii). Throughout the interviews,
the women emphasized their commitment to their respective communities
and expressed feelings of solidarity and unity. Some women, like Jocelyn,
the community educator from New York City, explained how the "foundation of my calling" in AIDS activism was the loved ones who were dying
and the duty she felt to educate people about their risks for HIV infection.
Sandy, a vice president of community development at a New York City-based
nonprofit, explains why she addressed AIDS: "Why AIDS? I don't know
I had a choice; I don't know I had a choice. It's a ministry." Using similar
religious overtones about community outreach and solidarity, Roxsan, a peer
educator from Dallas, explained, "I feel that God called me. . . . Back then

[when she became involved in AIDS activism work], in 2000, navigating the system was so difficult and I learned how to do it, so I felt it was a sin if I don't teach others how to do it, how to advocate for themselves."

Many of these activists explained that the duty they felt to address HIV rested in their desire to prevent what happened to themselves or to their loved ones—i.e., HIV infection—from happening to other individuals. Virginia, a 50-year-old AIDS educator who lives and works in Philadelphia, describes how she became involved in AIDS activism:

> *The primary reason why I got involved is I am, actually, I am a woman living with the virus. The second primary reason is because I have a sister who lost her fight to an AIDS-related illness back in the early '80s. So, you know, losing her and the way she, you know, the services that were not there for her just inspired me to make sure that . . . that I would be there at the table to make sure that when it comes to services, that what people need for HIV and AIDS, that they receive.*

Tara, a 59-year-old executive director of a women-centered nonprofit organization in Oakland, explains: "I first became aware of and involved in the AIDS issue years, and years, and years ago, but I wouldn't say that I was an activist until, you know, it struck home, and my brother contracted HIV. Then I became much more involved. And I think that's almost always the case." Tara later explains, "You know, there's a saying that 'the personal is political,' and I think that that is probably very much true. When things impact us personally, we take a look at it and, you know, then may be inspired to become involved in educating or shifting the power dynamics around the issue that we care about." The women discussed the realization that what impacted them also impacted others, and this created feelings of solidarity where they felt obligated, or "called," to care for other community members.

Feelings of community solidary motivated the women in our study to organize. According to Gilkes (2001) and Collins (2000), Black women derive their sense of identity from their communities, where they identify with other community members and their struggles. Gilkes (2001) and Collins (2000) also suggest that Black women center their communities' survival and are emotionally attached to their communities. As a result, they find solidarity with their community members and mobilize to help them.

CONCLUSION

Research has shown that emotions are not only commonly experienced during social and political activism, but importantly, emotions also drive and direct this activism (Gould 2009). As such, emotions help inspire individuals for collective action and can help scholars better understand social activism (Gould 2009). In sum, "feeling and emotion are fundamental to political life, not in the sense that they overtake reason and interfere with deliberative processes, as they are sometimes disparagingly construed to do, but there is an affective dimension to the processes and practices that make up 'the political,' broadly defined" (Gould 2009, 3).

This chapter used a womanist theoretical framework to examine the emotions that influence AIDS activism among Black women in the United States: love and compassion, anger and frustration, and feelings of solidarity and community. In her research on emotions and the ACT UP movement, Gould (2009) notes that shame and love led to the collective feelings of anger and frustration that initiated AIDS activism work and group solidarity; in turn, these feelings led to the ACT UP movement and organization. While this current study also finds that love, anger, and solidarity helped motivate these activists, this data shows that love appears to be at the core of the activism work of these women. Unlike in Gould's (2009) research, shame not only did not motivate our respondents, it was not even mentioned or expressed by the women in our study.

Womanism considers the unique ways Black women experience oppression, and how this oppression influences their identity formation and their response to social issues. Using a womanist framework, respondents in the study recognized that racism, homophobia, sexism, and classism are inherent in the response to HIV in Black communities and how this helped motivate their work. The women showed love, compassion, and care for their communities and their anger and frustration were rooted in their love for their communities. These feelings demonstrate how "othermothering" and community care are parts of the culture of Black women (Collins 2000; Gilkes 2001). The women felt love and compassion and recognized inequities that were inherent in the response to AIDS in their communities. These feelings led to the anger and frustration they expressed. This love and anger further led to feelings of solidarity and of community care among the activists, which fueled their activism work and desire to promote change within their communities.

Chapter Five

Education and Social Change

The previous chapter examined how emotions motivated the women in our study. The activists' love of themselves, love of community, and the pain of watching their community members die from a preventable illness helped motivate their AIDS activism. While emotions inspired personal feelings that enabled social action, AIDS knowledge empowered activists to envision solutions to broader social problems.

Multiple inequities, such as racism (Mackenzie 2013; Cohen 1999), sexism (Berger 2010; Ingram and Hutchinson 2000), and homophobia (Fullilove et al. 1990) impact AIDS rates within Black communities. Given that womanism privileges storytelling as its central epistemological framework, the knowledge production process, and knowledge in itself, are modes of resistance against social inequities. For example, the activists understood that there were community-specific modes of knowledge transmission that facilitated the expansion of AIDS information and education within their communities; similarly, the activists also understood that AIDS knowledge, AIDS facts, and educational materials play important roles in reducing AIDS rates. As a result, we apply womanism as a framework to understand how Black women AIDS activists posit strategies to mollify the AIDS epidemic in their communities and to reduce health inequities.

MEDICAL KNOWLEDGE AND BLACK COMMUNITIES

Muvuka et al. (2020) suggest health literacy or "health knowledge" bridges gaps between health providers and individuals. Muvuka et al. (2020) assume that when individuals have access to health knowledge, they are more likely to take preventative measures as well as to seek treatment for negative health outcomes. This framework can be applied to sexually-transmitted infections (STI) and HIV prevention education, including producing STI and AIDS information and knowledge (Rikard et al. 2012).

Public health has demonstrated that Black communities have lower access to AIDS knowledge for multiple reasons, including issues of stigma (Herek and Capitanio 1999), persistent conspiracy theories (Klonoff and Landrine 1999; Bogart and Thorburn 2005), religion (Sutton and Parks 2013), racism (Thomas and Quinn 1991), and other institutional factors (Cohen 1999; Dalton 1989). Within Black communities, AIDS stigma has affected how HIV-positive members perceive themselves (Cohen 1999, Harris 2010), but, importantly, this stigma has presented barriers to communal support and access to medical care. Furthermore, given their history of being the target of medical racism and experimentation, many within Black communities have often produced internal narratives that situate themselves as targets of governmental experimentation by reasoning that the government deploys AIDS as a means of regulating Black communities (Klonoff and Landrine 1999; Bogart and Thorburn 2005). As a result of medical racism and experiences of discrimination (Friedman 2009; Newman et al. 2008) and conspiracy theories (Brooks et al. 2018; Ojikutu et al. 2020), HIV prevention efforts, such as the use of PrEP (Ojikutu et al. 2020), have often been met with skepticism within Black communities.

Finally, there are internal dynamics within Black communities that prevent the spread of AIDS knowledge. For example, homophobia contributes to AIDS stigma and prevents major cultural institutions within Black communities, such as the Black Church, from distributing AIDS information (Fullilove et al. 1990; Harris 2010). Likewise, sexism affects AIDS knowledge and sexual practices within Black communities. Some of the ways in which sexism has impacted Black women and AIDS knowledge include a lack of autonomy over condom use (King and Hunter 2004; Ford et al. 2007), sexual norms (Stephens and Phillips 2005; Stephens and Few 2007) and an over-regulation of Black women's sexualities (Wagstaff et al. 1995; Wingood and DiClemente 1998). Finally, structural and systematic racism has made Black communities vulnerable to AIDS because public health efforts did not initially target Black communities, especially at the onset of the AIDS epidemic (Smith et al. 2005). These issues, rooted in systematic and structural racism, reduced access to AIDS public health efforts in Black communities (Yancy 2020; Bibbins-Domingo 2020). These are many of the same barriers that impact the experiences that Blacks have with other health issues, including, more recently, COVID-19 (Chandler et. al 2021).

WOMANISM, KNOWLEDGE PRODUCTION, AND HIV KNOWLEDGE

Womanism epistemologically encapsulates knowledge, the knowledge production process, marginality, and activism within its central tenets. Multiple Black scholars have described how knowledge generation can affirm Black experiences, especially Black women's experiences (hooks 1981; Collins 2000). For example, Collins (2002) documented how White men's experiences have dominated academia while negating the experiences of Black women. While womanist thought acknowledges that Black women's experiences have been historically underrepresented, womanism also acknowledges how the modes of knowledge transmission, such as storytelling and narrative, can empower Black communities. Given their origins in Afrocentric womanist thought and African oral traditions, these forms of epistemological transmission provide a culturally specific vernacular that contributes to overarching motifs within Black communities, including self-empowerment, community support, and spirituality (Phillips 2006; Douglas 2018). Researchers have examined this form of knowledge transmission in a wide variety of settings including nursing (Banks-Wallace 1998; 2000), pedagogy (Beauboeuf-Lafontant 2002; 2005), rhetoric (Hamlet 2000), therapy (Williams 2000), literary analysis (Ogunyemi 1985), social work (Carlton-LaNey 1999; 2001), media analyses (Pellerin 2012), and religion (Floyd-Thomas 2006).

In the context of AIDS activism and the spread of HIV and AIDS knowledge, womanist frameworks have been applied to understanding how community care (McLane-Davison 2016) and leadership (Smith-Ireland 2018) impacted the spread of AIDS knowledge. Other scholarship studied this participation and addressed how Black women AIDS activists seek to empower their communities through positions as community caretakers (Cloy 2016) and through spiritual engagement (Chambers 2018); however, these studies did not explicitly apply a womanist lens.

AIDS KNOWLEDGE AND SOCIAL CHANGE

Our study participants addressed how AIDS information can contribute to social change. All but one respondent described education's prominent role in AIDS activism. Peggy, a 57-year-old Denver-based consultant, explains, "I think education is an important step. I think prevention messages, written and verbally given, are important. I think follow-up to STI treatment is important." While broadly the respondents identified a lack of education as a key component of AIDS transmission, the women in our study had specific ideas for how prevention education should work. Crystal, a board member of the Southern AIDS Coalition, summarized:

> *Our anchor service is testing—knowing your status, making it accessible, available; reducing stigma so that people will get tested and know their status; integrating it into normalizing it; routine. And educating about what you do now and what you should do in the future if you don't want to be infected. And within that, we end up identifying and serving people living with HIV.*

Among other factors, Crystal mentioned that knowledge about status, access to AIDS testing, and the alleviation of stigma should be at the forefront of empowering the community.

Thus, the women essentially focused on three main areas of social change: knowing AIDS information, using peer groups to deploy this information, and expanding institutional access to HIV and AIDS knowledge.

AIDS Knowledge

Respondents described how knowledge about sexual behaviors, practices, and risk factors were paramount to HIV prevention. For example, Juliet, a 52-year-old AIDS activist, emphasized condom use: "You need women to use condoms. Use some kind of protection. You need women to understand. Just because you think you are in a monogamous relationship doesn't mean that you are, because if that was the case, we wouldn't have all of these married women infected." Likewise, Jennifer, a 54-year-old activist from Baton Rouge, noted how both men and women should use condoms: "Well, first off, I think they should have more condoms. Like some of the women are saying, 'Oh, he don't want to wear condoms. It don't feel right.' And you know, you know, so I say, 'Hey, look, that's female condoms.' You know. More female condoms being given out . . . [we are] educating people." Thus, both women emphasized condom use as part of education, but especially female condoms.

In addition, activists also mentioned knowledge of risk factors, like Isabella, a 41-year-old in Los Angeles, who noted:

> *The ideal tactics to address AIDS/HIV? I think just having a universal message and not so targeted on individual risk groups or populations. . . . It would talk about if you were having unprotected sex, whether it's vaginal or anal or oral, and if you are unaware of your status and your partner's status . . . you can be at risk. . . . [I]f you're getting tattoos outside of a reputable tattoo parlor, you are at risk. If you are using drugs, whether it's snorting, whether you're . . . maybe you're up in, like, Hollywood Hills at a party and you're snorting drugs behind somebody, that can put you at risk.*

Thus, the activists emphasized that their communities needed to understand specific risk factors that spread HIV and AIDS.

Peer Knowledge

While some of the women primarily highlighted knowledge surrounding AIDS, nine respondents stressed the importance of peers in Black communities spreading this AIDS knowledge. Our respondents believe that peer education involves the art of storytelling and emphasizing personal testimony. Shanice, a 59-year-old motivational speaker from New York, explains,

> *Well I don't sugarcoat anything. Sometimes, you know, they say you do. I don't. Like I said, I tell people, and I have the virus so I've been called on the carpet. The reason for peer education was to let people know that number one, they're not alone; number two, the person that's educating you has the virus. There's a lot of supervisors that feel that you just gotta educate them; you don't have to tell them [about your HIV status]. I don't mind telling them, especially when they ask you, "How do you know so much? How do you know this?" I tell them, "Look, I got the virus," you know? "I'm going through the same thing or maybe worse than you are. Don't tell me I don't know what I'm talking about." So, I, . . . to be truthful and to be honest, you know, and like I said, if I don't know something . . . I don't know everything. But you gotta be truthful and you gotta be honest and you don't talk down to them and you don't use large words that you can't spell anyway. I always ask . . . I try not to get too personable, but I'm always open after each group or meeting, or each when I speak or testimony, if anyone would want to come to me. I have my own personal business cards that I pass out. I tell them, "You can call me."*

Shanice provides a complex account of how her personal experiences with HIV can lend credibility to the information she provides. In this account, she explains that she is able to help others because her information is considered reliable as she lives with the virus herself. Additionally, she mentions that her message is based on honesty and truthfulness. Shanice also communicates in a way that is understandable and relatable because she mentions that her message "doesn't use large words you can't spell anyways." This is important because language can impact how audiences receive messages, highlighting Shanice's understanding of her target audience. Additionally, other women emphasized the role of covering information to address HIV stigma in Black communities. For example, Estelle, a 43-year-old case manager from North Carolina, explained,

> *We're going to have to just continue to get out there and speaking to people and hopefully with the information that we're sharing about the virus . . . It will help*

to reduce [HIV rates]. But at this point, all we can do is to continue in those great efforts that we've been doing and just hoping that more people will begin to take heed to the messages that are given.

However, this notion of "getting out there" had a lot to do with identifying stigma and working with major institutions that impact Black communities, namely the Black Church. Fifty-eight-year-old Brianna, an activist and motivational speaker from South Carolina, explains,

Well, the first step is to help eliminate the stigma. I mean, because of the stigma, people don't talk about it and if you're not talking about it, it's hard to educate or make it a household awareness when it's still hush-hush, taboo, and you know, we don't talk about those things. So, I think elimination of stigma is top priority. And then being able to dispel myths and educate on, how this disease is, is how you are infected. You know, the modes of transmission.

To dispel these myths, according to 60-year-old Milwaukee-based health project coordinator Lanetta, activists initiate a frank discussion around HIV prevention. Lanetta described,

I think, making it so that gay people are not marginalized and can be open and seek help just like any other, like someone who has chicken pox or athlete's foot or something like that. You know, you'd never be embarrassed about going to the doctor and saying, "I think I have athlete's foot." But going and saying, you know, "I'm a gay man, and I think I might be HIV-infected," or, you know, in this stage or that stage. People are not comfortable doing that. And you know, their families and everything.

To alleviate the stigma regarding AIDS and structurally marginalized sexual identities, the respondents wanted to initiate discussions related to health and identity. The women identified several places, including the Black Church, where these conversations should occur. Ena, 66-year-old founder of a social advocacy organization in Oakland, suggests,

Well, like I said earlier, doing the community forums, us talking with each other, having one-on-one [conversations]. The Church. Making sure that if your church doesn't have an AIDS ministry, to talk to them about AIDS ministry. Getting tested—tested, tested, tested—and making sure that if you get where the, if you're an African American woman and you get with a new relationship, that most of you guys get tested and get tested again, before you have unprotected sex.

Shay, a 56-year-old peer educator from South Carolina, also notes the need for more church involvement in AIDS education. Shay explained, "We need more people to get involved in [providing AIDS education]. And I'm talking about outside resources, such as our ministers and people of that nature. Where people tend to listen to. You know? They talk about other illnesses, but a lot of them don't talk about the HIV virus."

While the respondents described how AIDS information needed to circulate within religious institutions, others, like Tara, a 59-year-old executive director of an AIDS nonprofit said,

> *I think that women who are HIV-positive have a very important role in—particularly in an African American community—in reaching out to other African American women who may be experiencing all the other social issues that make them much more susceptible to contracting HIV. So, we need to have peers in the domestic violence shelters. We need to have peers talking to, the best that we can, partners of incarcerated men. We need to have peers working with the agencies that provide addiction services. You know, in my dream, we would be interacting and collaborating with all of these different people.*

In addition to the Black Church, Tara suggested that activists should collaborate with other institutions that cater to more vulnerable populations. Thus, peer groups were perceived as instrumental to spreading AIDS knowledge and information.

Values and Knowledge

The respondents described how teaching values is important in HIV prevention. For example, Sandy, a 48-year-old activist who works as the vice president of community development in New York City, explains, "It's about us going back to some of the basics. It's about instilling values on our young people, teaching them to love themselves before they love someone, [and] not looking for love in all the wrong places. It's about getting our leaders to have uniform conversations and find sort of talking points that [are] for more real-life conversations." While emphasizing peer mentorship, she also stresses the importance of self-love. Echoing this notion, 53-year-old Betty, who works as a peer educator in Maryland, suggests AIDS educators work at "building up their [clientele's] self-esteem and again, teaching them how to protect themselves. Don't just listen to the story of 'I love you' stories; always protect yourself. Never depend on a man to have these things; you carry these things for yourself." Likewise, in the context of describing that HIV is preventable, 50-year-old Dorothy, an AIDS advocate from Oakland, emphasizes that women should "respect and educate themselves." Thus, for these activists, protection centers around self-worth, self-empowerment, and self-respect.

Womanism addresses how these women reconcile their community-specific knowledge with their ability to marshal social change. We emphasize womanism's notion of self-empowerment because it provides a framework by which Black women position themselves as agents of social change rather than victims of social inequities. This framework posits that Black women occupy a structurally marginalized position, and, in addition to basing their identities on activism, these women develop knowledge that resists dominant power structures through affirming spiritualist belief systems, communal support, self-empowerment, and storytelling. Social scientific literature has applied womanism in the arenas of pedagogy (Beauboeuf-Lafontant 2002; 2005), therapy (Williams 2000), nursing (Taylor 1998; Shambley-Ebron and Boyle 2006), and other forms of "interventions" that have called for reframing knowledge to "better suit" structurally marginalized audiences, including Black communities within the AIDS epidemic. These findings extend womanist frameworks because respondents find empowerment through AIDS education, and they believe this information prevents AIDS within Black communities. This notion is similar to how womanist scholars argue that knowledge generation produces both empowerment and liberation.

Additionally, in line with womanist thought, the modes of knowledge transmission are relevant to community support and the eradication of AIDS. Underscoring the importance of peer mentorship, the women in our study mentioned that "trust" between individuals within Black communities enables people to feel "less embarrassed" when seeking AIDS information. This then places a greater emphasis on community support because peer education can mollify AIDS stigma as well as create stronger representation within Black communities.

ADDRESSING INSTITUTIONAL ACCESS

In addition to being informed about sexual behaviors, practices, and risk factors, the activists discussed the importance of access to different social institutions. Tammy, a 37-year-old sex educator from Philadelphia, described "education, testing, access to care, [and] affordable, accessible medication" as the most important components of HIV prevention. According to 51-year-old New York City-based activist Jasmine,

> *The most important step is [to] continue to provide education . . . because the more people we get tested, the better off the health of the community will be. And then from there, we'll be able to go forward. And our community is sick and in poor health and the people living in the community are sick. . . . So, the more*

people we get tested, that show their status, that were able to engage in health care, the better off we'll be.

Similarly, Roxsan, 65-year-old peer educator from Dallas, noted that testing can be increased by increasing ongoing programming and providing additional support services. Roxsan asserted,

We have to reduce stigma. We have to increase those tested, you have to decrease infection, and you have to increase those in care. Those four things are the four things that the National AIDS Strategy stresses. And so, everything we do should be something that adds toward those things. And we shouldn't just wait once a year in June, which is the HIV Testing Month, that you decide, "Let's get everybody tested!" I mean, some things should be more ongoing.

In addition to lacking access to testing, AIDS activist Beatrice, a 56-year-old AIDS advocate from New York City who runs a health service organization, describes how many within Black communities face numerous obstacles while navigating social institutions:

Well, I think it's, first of all, actually letting Black people know the extent of the disease within the community, right? That would be the first step, I think, and assisting them in how to maneuver the particular systems that are in place to help them because people have no idea. I even look at even when you go to any sort of hospital or any sort of institution, it's how do you maneuver in that institution? How do you know, get to see the doctor, see the nurse, see the case manager without actually going bonkers about how to figure it out, right? So, it's about access; I think it's access to education, I think it's access to health care, I think it's access to housing, it's drugs, child care, all sort of things.

When describing how Black communities need to understand the extent of the disease, similar to Beatrice, the activists emphasize that many are simply unable to navigate healthcare institutions. In addition to ongoing access to resources (e.g., AIDS testing), the respondents described how a lack of representation and thorough sex education impeded the spread of AIDS knowledge within Black communities.

Representation

The women in our study described how representation is important for Black communities and their access to AIDS services. Fifty-one-year-old Roxsan, an AIDS educator from Dallas, described how access must be culturally relevant, "Again, to really develop each of the prevention programs that speak the language of the people they are working with that are culturally sensitive that comes from the strength that the community brings to these prevention programs. Not dictating, you know, like you need this more like you have a voice we honor your voice as a Black woman." She further explained,

> *Tell us what you need to be able to negotiate safer sex and see we can model programs but that also means on a higher level, not a higher level but another level, really disrupting the cultural norms in the communities changing the way people think about women, men, sex, drugs, alcohol, power. A lot got to be disruptive in order to address the rate of infection. It's really about stepping out in a very brave way and really not wanting people staying in the same box. Thus, access includes both access to programs, but also programs that are culturally relevant to Black communities.*

In addition to Roxsan's emphasis on the importance of culturally relevant language, 49-year-old Ruby, an activist from San Diego, explained how this representation motivates her by

> *knowing that there's a face out there like mine helping to remove the stigma. A little girl [on TV] prompted me to be more active. You know, when I saw her on TV, I said wait a minute. She's seven years old. She's telling the world she's HIV-positive. She was a little Black girl from the projects . . . that pushed me to want to be more of an advocate for HIV. If she could do it, I know I could do it. And let the world see that we're living with [HIV].*

For Ruby, a visual representation of someone with HIV helped her connect to others with AIDS and inspired her to serve as an advocate. As the activists spoke of access to culturally relevant education, several other respondents focused on institutions within formal educational settings, especially sex education.

Access to Sexual Education

Respondents explained that sexual education in schools increases understandings of HIV prevention. Tracy, 31-year-old activist from Philadelphia, noted that basic information of how HIV is spread must be addressed by

> *comprehensive sex education in the school. So, if as a society we're making any changes towards what occurs, you need to lay that seed. And I think if you have that education in the schools, people have a better idea of what's going on with their bodies, how what they do will have an impact on their body. Then as a society, as they're older, they'll have the tools to make the decisions from there. . . . But I don't even think we're giving anyone the proper tools to make the better decisions. It's just kind of, "We'll give a class for two days in eighth grade," but something may have already occurred by then, so the tools aren't*

really there or in place. So as a society, I think it really started with providing that proper education for them but, even that's difficult, because if you look at the schools now and everything, they're cutting, then that'll go, that'll open another door of issues. So, I mean, I think it's an idealistic approach to it, but I think it's important.

Even though Tracy acknowledges this as a lofty goal, Grace, a 46-year-old activist and medical case manager from the New Orleans, agreed that "comprehensive" sex education is key. Grace explains,

People think that comprehensive sexuality education is just talking about sex, but in that model, you talk about positive body image. You talk about differences in body image, you know, in the ways bodies are made. You talk about setting goals. You talk about all these things that truly impact a person, and then that does away with some of those social determinants of health. If a person is well-educated, then you know what? Lack of education goes out the window. If a person is making enough money, then poverty goes out the window. You know, so it's things we can do to educate our youth so that 10, 15 years from now, we're not still having the same conversation.

Dana, a 59-year-old activist from Philadelphia, pushed for more educational opportunities, in general, for adults: "I think that what's important for us to do better, is to push more for adult education that's not even AIDS specific. To push more for adult education because what keeps people from fighting is that they think they're not smart enough to fight, because they know they have to fight systems." Therefore, these activists stressed that Black communities needed to create access by reforming sexual education targeting their communities.

Finally, the women in our study also called for addressing problems that are adjacent to the AIDS crisis, including poverty, comprehensive sex education, and domestic violence. Womanist thought calls for a recognition of broader social problems that are not exclusive to the plight of Black women. By addressing adjacent issues to the AIDS epidemic, womanism aptly helps us better understand the approach the women in our study use to frame education in their communities.

In order to address gaps between Black communities and public health institutions, the activists described how representation and sex education play key roles in how to better connect health information with structurally marginalized communities. Current literature addresses a "knowledge gap" within Black communities and calls for education as a means of addressing AIDS (Muvuka et al. 2020). This literature also posits questions around sexual autonomy (Johnson et al. 1992; Exner et al. 2003) and describes how HIV prevention is stymied by stigma (Herek and Capitanio 1999), conspiracy theories (Klonoff and Landrine 1999; Bogart and Thorburn 2005), the prison industrial complex (Fogel and Beylyea 1999), and several other institutional factors (Harris 2010; Cohen 1999). While these factors are present within Black communities, these branches of literature have not explained how Blacks address this "knowledge gap" within their communities. Particularly, literature highlights how the sexism that Black women often experience in these communities, including stereotypes and power inequities, coincide with their higher HIV infection rates (Campbell and Soeken 1999; Fullilove et al. 1990).

We find that, while Black women are vulnerable to HIV, they also develop community-specific strategies to combat the virus. Specifically, the data presented shows that Black women AIDS activists understand both problems and solutions to the epidemic, and they mobilize to create change within their own communities. By deploying AIDS information, Black women relay information to their own communities and address institutional factors not centered in larger public health campaigns.

CONCLUSION

The women in our study deployed medical knowledge as a means of empowerment and called for education as the primary means of social change. They advocated for the spread of HIV educational information and suggested that targeting cultural institutions, such as the Black Church, was also important in spreading HIV and AIDS knowledge. To a lesser degree, the respondents discussed how values were important in spreading information, but, ultimately, the women described how representation efforts, including creating culturally relevant and comprehensive sex education programs and resources, were important for social change.

Research suggests that Black communities have limited access to AIDS education, thereby exacerbating Black communities' vulnerability to HIV (Muvuka et al. 2020). In addition, Black women are frequently portrayed as victims of HIV (Wagstaff et al. 1995; Wingood and DiClemente 1998), specifically because of stereotypes and other forms of inequities. However, womanist frameworks emphasize Black women's agency in resisting structural marginalization and situate them as agents of social change. Importantly, womanism emphasizes Black women's abilities to develop knowledge and modes of knowledge dissemination in order to combat social inequities. The literature has highlighted how researchers have applied womanist frameworks to address the "knowledge gaps" between structurally marginalized communities and dominant structures (Beauboeuf-Lafontant 2002; 2005)

The women in our study privilege "knowing" AIDS information and being able to spread this knowledge within Black communities. Specifically, they highlight how fostering greater trust within Black communities and their institutions alleviates stigma and prevents HIV transmission. Furthermore, the activists' responses described how addressing institutional factors, such as underrepresentation and comprehensive sexual education, can address the AIDS crisis in Black communities. This data demonstrates how womanism aptly describes how Black women generate and deploy knowledge for communal support, thus reducing the spread of AIDS within Black communities.

Chapter Six

Conclusion

This book focuses on AIDS activism among Black women. A key aspect of this text is its emphasis on womanism and its contributions to analyzing the lives and experiences of Black women activists. Both Black feminist thought and intersectionality, respectively, provide an epistemological and analytical lens that center the experiences of Black women. Nevertheless, womanist thought differs from Black feminist thought and intersectionality as it places an emphasis on all structurally marginalized individuals and groups, not just Black women. Womanism also focuses on interlocking structures of oppression and self-empowerment, spirituality, and social change. We applied a womanist theoretical framework to better understand what encourages AIDS activism among Black women. We analyzed 36 interviews with Black women AIDS activists from around the United States and then organized the data gathered from their responses into major themes.

First, we found Black women AIDS activists negotiated their racial and gendered identities. We found that given the history of how Black women engage in communal support and serve as community caretakers, Black women AIDS activists organized because they acted to protect and to support their communities from AIDS. As a result, these women did not identify with notions of mainstream feminism for two reasons. The activists felt that feminism overlooked racism as an axis of inequity. Also, feminism avoided discussions of how the intersections of class, race, gender, sexuality, and other structures of domination impact Black communities afflicted with AIDS.

We located Black women AIDS activists within their religious and spiritual contexts. We examined how Black communities have culturally revolved around Black churches and religion. Nonetheless, the activists identified themselves as spiritual instead of religious because of social inequities that permeate within Black churches, namely sexism and homophobia. Thus, while there were traces of religiosity in their belief systems, the respondents largely abandoned notions of religion in favor of spirituality-based belief systems.

We then discussed the role of emotions, such as anger and love, as an impetus for organizing. While these respondents had goals of eradicating AIDS within their communities, they personalized the impact of the AIDS epidemic because it affected their loved ones. They expressed "anger" and frustration toward social inequities and expressed love for their communities. Thus, we found that these women prioritized their emotions because these emotions empowered them toward social action.

Finally, we examined how the respondents addressed gaps in medical knowledge. While AIDS disproportionately affects Black communities, public health highlights gaps in AIDS knowledge. The respondents overwhelmingly posited education as the main suggestion for change within their communities and focused mainly on condom-use education as well as the culturally specific sites of knowledge deployment. As such, they argue that education is not only a key mechanism of social change, but, also, specified types of education and sites of knowledge deployment.

THEORETICAL IMPLICATIONS

As mentioned before, Black feminist thought, intersectionality, and womanism center the experiences of structurally marginalized women as sites of epistemology. Black feminist thought and womanist epistemologies focus on the experiences of Black women. In chapter 1, we highlighted the similarities between Black feminist thought, womanism, and intersectionality and how they center Black women's experiences. However, there are also several theoretical limitations. While addressing theoretical gaps presented by White, Eurocentric academic, and feminist discourse, Black feminist thought and intersectionality failed to examine the interlocking experience of inequity among structurally marginalized individuals who are not Black women. Intersectionality and Black feminist thought highlight the experiences of Black women and did so through providing an analytical lens which explores how interlocking identities structured social relations. Intersectionality also posited a methodological framework in order to understand the experience of interlocking identities. However, these two frameworks focus on the experiences of Black women and theorize interlocking systems of racism and sexism as mechanisms of social constraint. From womanist frameworks, Black women and other structurally marginalized individuals are empowered to both recognize and combat constraints of multiple inequities, such as racism, sexuality, poverty, homophobia, and classism. Womanist frameworks also hold that spirituality intertwines with social justice and bridges theory (epistemology) and praxis.

In addition, as a framework, womanism has both American and Africana iterations. In its African iteration, Africana womanism incorporates African spiritualism into its understanding of social relations, especially as it highlights feminism's Eurocentric biases (Reed 2001). For example, Africana womanism attempts to center African women's experiences, but also establishes communal relationships between women and men as it argues that spiritually, women and men are connected within "the whole" and "the divine" (Hudson-Weems 2019). This notion of the "whole" frames Africana womanist understandings of social institutions (within marriage and family, for example), where communities and families, rather than individuals, are interconnected (Hudson-Weems 2019). Thus, Africana womanism provided the spiritualist and theoretical underpinnings for American womanist frameworks.

In line with womanist thought, the women in our study noted that in addition to combating racism, they also knew that they needed to dismantle other structures of inequity for social liberation. This helped serve as the impetus for their mobilization. In addition, some of the respondents were HIV-positive; as a result, their emotions likely affected how they mobilized against the epidemic.

Likewise, spirituality played a key role in the activism work of the women in our study. A majority of the activists described how they were raised in deeply religious communities, but many left these communities because of sexism and homophobia. Spiritualist systems emphasize a nonhierarchical belief in a higher power or God; this enabled respondents to mobilize against AIDS within their communities. Womanism highlights spirituality as crucial to its framework, whereas Black feminist thought and intersectionality do not emphasize spirituality within the experiences of those who face structural marginalization.

Furthermore, emotions such as anger and love motivated the respondents to mobilize. Womanist frameworks, especially Afrocentric iterations of the framework, privilege community and emphasize communal survival. Womanism then situates these feelings as both epistemology and praxis. As epistemology, womanism's emphasis on communal survival impacts emotions and helps us understand how study participants framed their experiences around their emotions. This then differs between Black feminist thought and intersectionality because these frameworks highlight the *experience* of inequity, not necessarily the *emotions* that result from said social inequities.

Finally, the respondents also posited suggestions for social change. By suggesting education as a means of change, the activists demonstrate their capacity for agency and empowerment, and how they deploy culturally specific information to address inequities within their communities. However, while the information is culturally specific, the information highlights interlocking inequities that affect Black communities. From a womanist framework, while the women understood that AIDS disproportionately affects their communities, they also recognized interlocking forms of social inequities. Furthermore, Black feminist thought and intersectionality recognize inequity as it specifically affects Black women; these frameworks do not posit solutions to addressing social inequities.

While Black feminist thought and intersectionality are commonly used when analyzing Black women's experiences, womanism explains Black women AIDS activists' experiences in a more nuanced way. Black feminist thought and intersectionality largely explain social inequities from Black women's perspectives, but fail to provide effective praxis. While these perspectives sometimes lend themselves to methodological interventions, they do not adequately prescribe frameworks for social change.

Womanism, on the other hand, is both epistemology and praxis. It is a multidimensional lens that encapsulates how Black women's experiences relate to their understandings of their spiritualties, understandings of their own race and gender identities, and understandings of their relation to the Black Church. Womanist lenses also encapsulate understandings of multiple axes of social inequities as sites of social control, understandings of mobilization against social inequities, understandings of love and anger, understandings of culturally specific strategies for social change, understandings of privileging emotions as valid epistemological sites, and understandings of agency/empowerment.

CONTRIBUTIONS TO PUBLIC HEALTH/AIDS ACTIVISM

We find that public health efforts need to account for how sociocultural factors impact individuals' ability to mobilize against health issues and how health activists center their mobilization efforts. Based on our data, we provide several suggestions for AIDS activism and public health.

First, our data have demonstrated that historical underpinnings of community context shape forces that enable activists to organize around health issues. As a result, these contextual factors, racial identity commitment, and gendered cultural demands affected how the respondents mobilized. This means that public health must manage how it markets health information to structurally marginalized communities. Likewise, public health must also be aware that the particular ideologies that attempt to mollify disparities (e.g., feminism) might also negatively impact how people mobilize against health inequities, as was the case with respondents' shift away from mainstream feminism.

Second, cultural ideologies and structures heavily influence activist efforts. We found that even though the respondents shied away from the Black Church and religion itself, belief structures were still important in their mobilization efforts. Thus, AIDS activism and public health could continue to underscore the role of both religion and spirituality in relation to how individuals mobilize against AIDS.

Third, activism and mobilization efforts are not rational processes. Our data describes how the activists mobilized around not only culturally constructed understandings of illness and disease, but also how they mobilized around "goal-oriented and "emotion-driven" incentives. In other words, while the respondents had culturally and historically specific reasons why they mobilized, emotions were key factors in the process of mobilization. The women "hated" their oppression as much as they "loved" their communities, and these emotions drove their actions. Thus, public health and AIDS activism should work to better understand community members' feelings and emotions when they attempt to create messaging for a particular campaign.

Finally, public health and AIDS activism should underscore the importance of activist experiences within their own communities and should develop their campaigns based on their suggestions. Our data finds that activists understand the factors that affected their community's struggles with the epidemic, and they also posited suggestions that were culturally specific to their communities.

FUTURE DIRECTIONS

While our study has thoroughly examined the various processes and explanations for how and why Black women engage in AIDS activism, there were limitations. Methodologically, while our data attempted to undertake a theoretical sample, many of the women in our sample were highly educated and served in leadership positions. As such, our respondents, on the whole, inhabited social positions that are not representative of those who are less privileged; in essence, this could have impacted our data. Likewise, our understanding of womanism wholly applied to the experiences of cisgender Black women, and, as such, future work should examine how other structurally marginalized groups, especially other women of color and trans women of color, deploy womanist mobilization strategies and activism. Finally, this study can be used to further understand how Black women mobilize to address other pressing community challenges, such as COVID-19 and police brutality.

CONCLUSION

This book uses a womanist framework to examine AIDS activism among Black women in the U.S. and finds sociocultural and historically specific positions greatly impacted their reasons for mobilization and the experiences they have in their activism work. We also find that respondents deemphasized feminist understandings of social mobilization in favor of combating racial, economic, and other forms of inequity. Furthermore, our study suggests that spirituality and emotions affected how these women mobilized. Finally, the activists deployed suggestions—much of which were based on their personal experiences and interactions—in order to address AIDS knowledge gaps within their communities.

This text argues that womanism aptly describes how Black women mobilize to address social problems in their respective communities. We argued that Black feminist thought and intersectionality, while important epistemological and analytical frameworks and tools, do not adequately describe the experiences of Black women AIDS activists. Instead, we find that womanism provides a better framework to explain how and why Black women mobilize, especially since both the women in our study and womanism as a framework underscore the importance of self-empowerment, interlocking structures of oppression, spirituality, and social mobilization.

Additionally, given these theoretical contributions, we are able to contribute to scholarship that explores how AIDS activists and public health officials can partner with community advocates to develop health messaging and social marketing campaigns that more specifically target and address community concerns. We posit that public health can emphasize the importance of context while addressing AIDS disparities within particular communities. We argue that cultural institutions, such as the Black Church, are important institutions within Black communities and that they are important places to raise AIDS awareness. We also suggest that public health campaigns should not underplay the role of emotions in activism efforts.

Public health researchers and officials should continue to consider the perspectives of community activists while developing health promotion campaigns and strategies. Black women have a long history of activism and community engagement, and, more than any other group, have vigorously worked to address the needs and concerns facing members of Black communities. It is vital that researchers and healthcare professionals not only study health disparities and social inequities in structurally marginalized groups, but that they listen to and actively engage with communities—working *with* them to address *their* concerns. By providing resources and funding, and by working with those who are both directly impacted by a particular issue (whether it be

HIV or some other social problem) and who have dedicated their lives to addressing community concerns, real, innovative, substantive, and sustainable change can take place. In addition, we urge researchers and social scientists to explore womanism as a theoretical and methodological framework when examining activism and community engagement among women of color, and in particular, among Black women.

Appendix A

Toward an Embodied Womanist Methodology

In this section, we examine the relationship between epistemology and methodology in order to expand upon womanist methodology. We begin our discussion with a brief overview of the main conceptual points that are highlighted in the book and discuss our findings. We will then reexamine some quotes and themes presented in the text to better examine intersectional epistemologies, womanist epistemologies, and how these epistemologies affect the development of research methodology. Given that we introduce intersectional and womanist epistemology in chapter 1, here, we focus on the theoretical and methodological implications of intersectional and womanist epistemologies.

In order to expand womanist methodologies, we build on "storytelling" as the main component of womanist methodology. In addition, based on our data, we include themes such as the individual identity, social structure, cultural/historical context, religion and spirituality, visceral embodiment, and culturally relevant epistemological framings. From these main components, we then highlight and explain six main principles of our method that we call "embodied womanism." We then discuss the implications and limitations of womanism as a methodological and theoretical framework.

TOWARD WOMANIST SOCIAL SCIENTIFIC METHODS

In the first chapter, we described how AIDS rates disproportionately impact Black communities and how Black women address this public health problem by mobilizing to address AIDS in their communities. We identified several structural and cultural factors that contribute to how and why Black communities continue to be negatively impacted by AIDS. We also introduced intersectional and womanist frameworks to explain how and why Black women mobilize against AIDS.

We identified five main themes from 36 interviews with Black women AIDS activists. These themes explain the varied motivations for AIDS activism among these women. We also found that study participants appeal to culturally specific modes of community survival as parts of their social mobilization strategy (chapter 2). A majority of the respondents appealed to a set of spiritualist values by often evoking an appeal to a higher spiritual power when engaging in AIDS activism as opposed to conforming to traditional religious values (chapter 3). We found that emotions, specifically anger and love, motivated the activists (chapter 4). Finally, the women advocated for Black religious leaders and comprehensive sex education programs to serve as vectors for educational solutions that address the AIDS crisis within their communities (chapter 5).

We concluded with an examination of the limitations of intersectionality in chapter 6. By explaining how Black women serve as caretakers within their communities and reject feminism as an identity, we find that Black women emphasize the collective struggles of their communities over their need to mobilize based on different aspects of their identity (e.g., their gender). The women in our study center their communal bonds and overtly tie their activism to their identity as Black women. In contrast, unlike womanist frameworks, intersectionality does not specifically emphasize these bonds and separates identity from activism. Intersectionality also does not highlight religion or spirituality as important aspects of one's identity. Finally, intersectionality does not address how storytelling affects how communities relay culturally specific messages. Rather, intersectionality is a tool employed by womanist and Black feminist theorists to better understand the impact that intersecting identities have on individuals and their oppressions.

Womanist epistemology best explains community mobilization in response to AIDS and provides a stronger methodological framework to understand Black women's AIDS activism. Intersectionality's epistemology affects how its theorists construct methodologies to study the social world and the experiences of structurally marginalized people. Mainly, intersectionality focuses on identifying nuances of one's social position and related outcomes, and, as such, affects how researchers collect data. Conversely, womanist epistemology centers Afrocentric notions of community-building where there is an emphasis on oral tradition, collective solidarity, and spiritualism that emphasizes the unity of the community. In its American iteration, womanism focuses on emphasizing these features by centralizing storytelling as the primary mode of communal knowledge transmission. As such, womanist methodologies in the social sciences emphasize these epistemological framings during the data collection process.

Thus, while we argue that womanist research methodologies address the limitations of intersectional methodologies, we also extend the logic of womanist epistemology in order to develop a nuanced framework that extends womanist methods. Based on our findings, we identify five main dimensions of womanist epistemology: storytelling and oral tradition, structurally marginalized communities and interlocking oppressions, spirituality and religiosity, emotions and embodied action, and knowledge and its production. Through these dimensions of womanist epistemology, we develop six main principles of social scientific research. We then address the benefits and limitations of these methodological principles within the context of existing womanist research methodologies.

INTERSECTIONALITY AND METHODOLOGY

In order to understand how womanist research methodologies offer a nuanced framework to better analyze the experiences of Black women and other structurally marginalized groups, we first examine how intersectionality's epistemology affects its methodology and intersectionality's limitations.

Chapter 1 describes intersectionality as a theoretical framework posited by Kimberlé Williams Crenshaw, Patricia Hill Collins, and other researchers who argue that individual identities and outcomes are shaped through a matrix of oppression (Collins 2002). Collins (2002) developed her methodological approaches based on this epistemology. She describes how White men have dominated academic knowledge production by emphasizing notions of objectivity and neutrality, and, in doing so, how they have controlled the valuation systems of particular forms of knowledge within academic institutions, mainly through valuing empirically based research that emphasizes rigorous research methodologies. Collins then explains how we must value the contributions of Black women's experiences by focusing on how they produce epistemology, which is often through creative endeavors, such as music, art, literature, or poetry. In other words, in order to address Eurocentric, racist, and sexist forms of knowledge production, Collins suggests that the academy value Black women's various forms of knowledge production, even if they fall outside of the contexts of conventional modes of academic knowledge production. Thus, Collins's reaction to her epistemological argument centers knowledge production discourse as both epistemology as well as methodology.

However, this framework has limitations. While researchers and activists have applied intersectionality for social justice, it is largely an analytical framework that essentially identifies specific struggles of specific groups, and, largely, intersectionality does not explicitly posit a framework of social change other than its ability to center the experiences of specific groups of individuals (e.g., Black women, Black heterosexual women, and Black lesbians who navigate x, y, and z). In this vein, intersectionality can be applied to center the experiences of a particular group, but it does not highlight how activism is inherently part of this group identity. As such, intersectionality privileges intersecting individual identities rather than explaining how individuals form ties within their communities.

INTERSECTIONAL METHODOLOGIES

Intersectional epistemologies lend themselves to developing intersectional methodologies, or practical methodological tools that are applied by social scientists to generate identity-based knowledge. Intersectional methodologies focus on developing singular-identity-based knowledge (e.g., Black women as singular identities). In intersectional research, for example, findings can only apply to the group in question rather than being able to extrapolate the data to other communities. For example, findings that apply to Black heterosexual women will not necessarily apply to the Black lesbian experience. Thus, when intersectionality-based theoretical framings are applied, researchers focus on the uniqueness of said identity, and sometimes this is done in comparison to other (dominant) groups in order to demonstrate inequity. Likewise, as a research methodology, intersectionality can also impact how data is collected. By applying specific techniques through interviewing methods, the researcher mainly attempts to understand the motivations of a particular group. Sometimes, intersectional methodologies can examine within-group variation rather than examining the group's relationship to its communities.

Epistemologically, intersectionality has been applied to focus on how different groups navigate various inequities. This framework has permeated into different aspects of social scientific research, including both qualitative and quantitative research methodologies (Harris and Bartlow 2015). In her analysis of interview questions, Bowleg (2008) posits different question types that can engage respondents and elicit information that incorporates various aspects of identity by asking direct questions about a respondent's race and gender, rank ordering the importance of different identity positions, and incorporating other ways of addressing the experiences of structurally marginalized groups. In addition, Bowleg (2008) has also argued that one can incorporate a similar system of rank ordering of identity importance in survey research.

Social scientific approaches to health and intersectional research can be useful to target specific experiences and outcomes as they document Black women and other structurally marginalized groups. However, these approaches are limited because they provide a cross-sectional approach to the study of marginalized experiences that highlight specific outcomes within specific moments in time. Likewise, intersectional methodologies do not examine Black women's history of community support and community ties. In addition, while intersectionality focuses on structurally marginalized individuals, the navigation of multiple identities, and structural outcomes, intersectionality does not necessarily examine intra-community ties as they relate to how structurally marginalized communities navigate social inequities. Similarly, while there is an emphasis on social outcomes, intersectional research neither methodologically focuses on the bonds of structurally marginalized communities, nor does it focus on how individuals resist inequity.

In contrast to intersectional research methodologies, womanist methodologies privilege storytelling and community networks. Womanist methodologies focus on how social scientists empirically apply womanist frameworks to collect data on Black women's experiences. Also, rather than simply being an analytical tool, womanism emphasizes how structurally marginalized individuals connect to other community members based on their experiences, and, from this connection, individuals are empowered. Ultimately, intersectionality's epistemological emphasis on identity produces several limitations for its usefulness as a methodology. This starkly contrasts to womanism's methodological strengths because womanism privileges storytelling as well as its relationship with community.

In sum, intersectionality-based methodologies reinforce their epistemological underpinnings in intersectional and Black feminist thought, and these methods also have limitations on the production of social scientific data. Based on womanist theory, womanist methods apply womanist thought and provide a stronger analysis for Black women's experiences, especially since they highlight storytelling and the community. However, while we offer womanist frameworks for examining the social world, our findings suggest that these womanist methodologies can be improved by offering additional metrics to womanist research methodologies and offering a "tool" that examines how Black women's experiences can be applied to engage in critical health research.

WOMANISM AND METHODOLOGY

In chapters 1 and 2, we explain womanism and its validation of Black women's cultural emphasis on storytelling, relationship to community building, spirituality, empowerment through community ties, modes of social change, and resistance against dominant structures. In its Afrocentric conception, Africana womanism centers the community bond by emphasizing social solidarity and unification through spiritualist principles and storytelling. As a derivation from Afrocentric womanist principles, American womanism has centered primarily on the following elements: storytelling, spirituality, empowerment, community solidarity, interconnectedness, and resistance to dominant structures. American womanism is based on lived and pragmatic experiences and on how Black communities emphasize community ties. Additionally, even though womanism was developed based on the experiences of Black women, a womanist framework can be applied to the experiences of *all* structurally marginalized individuals. Thus, womanism as an epistemology is more inclusive of all marginalized experiences, and it accounts for emotions and spirituality. This creates a contrast between intersectionality and womanism because intersectionality's main theoretical underpinnings suggest that it is an academic analytical tool meant to produce knowledge. Conversely, these underpinnings do not suggest that it is a framework that documents individual lived experiences as these experiences relate to structurally marginalized identity and community-building.

Especially highlighted in both its Afrocentric and American iterations, womanism has centered storytelling as its central tenet; thus, oral tradition and "storytelling" are the primary means through which scholars define womanist methods. For example, Walker (1994) suggests Black women's community experiences are embodied in their stories. Eventually, this emphasis on storytelling would permeate literary criticism and religious scripture interpretation via hermeneutical methodologies. In addition to being applied to literary criticism and religious hermeneutical interpretation, womanism was applied to the social sciences as a theoretical framing (as with our study) and an empirically based methodology, especially in the fields of education/pedagogy, nursing, health equity sciences, and psychology, where scholars have incorporated, for example, storytelling into their methodology. For example, Marr (2014) developed a womanist pedagogical practice that integrated storytelling in the classroom while some womanism-influenced psychology scholars (Williams 2000) integrated storytelling into therapy protocols for structurally marginalized groups.

In our study, we focused on furthering a womanist theoretical framework; however, methodologically, while we implicitly engaged in telling the stories of Black women AIDS activists, we did so through grounded theory methods, which focus on meaning-making and the (social) construction of individual stories (Glaser and Strauss 2017). Thus, from a grounded theory design, while the women in our study recount their experiences, it is not specifically through a distinct womanist framework, and this is indeed a methodological limitation. However, with our findings, we are able to develop a methodological framework that can impact the social scientific study of womanism.

While these approaches integrate womanism as methodology, we believe that our findings also address methodological limitations within empirically driven womanist research. For example, in a number of studies (Shambley-Ebron and Boyle 2006; Floyd-Thomas 2006), while there is an emphasis on Black communities, these studies are ahistorical and do not articulate the experience of Black communities within interlocking structures. Likewise, where some studies focus on religion (Lincoln and Mamiya 1990; Douglas 2018), these studies account for how Black communities negotiate spirituality as a mode of practice. Our study found that spirituality and religion are distinct concepts that have different appeals for many within Black communities, the interconnection between religiosity and spirituality, and the relevance of structural actors on Black individuals' spirituality. Thus, these current methodological approaches do not nuance their understandings of spirituality in the way they measure and account for spiritual dynamics. While womanist research has emphasized the practicality of Black women's experience, it does not consider metrics that examine structurally marginalized individuals, their communal bonds, and their physical outcomes (data presented in chapter 4). Finally, while womanist methodologies in social scientific research have demonstrated the impact of cultural authority, they do not nuance types of authorities and contexts that produce community-based knowledge within Black communities.

To address these limitations within womanist approaches in social scientific methodologies, we propose an empirically based methodology called the "embodied womanist methodology," which attempts to address these limitations based on the literature reviewed and data collected in chapters 1–5.

EXPANDING WOMANIST METHODOLOGICAL FRAMEWORKS THROUGH DATA

Our study demonstrated that Black women's AIDS activism is best understood through womanist principles. In chapters 2–5, we reviewed literature and presented data that suggest that womanism provides a better understanding of how Black women mobilize against AIDS. However, with these findings, we can also develop and expand womanist methodological frameworks in order to nuance future womanist empirical research.

Our study identified five main dimensions that can influence womanist data collection: 1) storytelling, 2) identifying relevant community structures, 3) locating spirituality and appealing to universal ethics, 4) identifying visceral and corporal embodiments, and 5) identifying epistemological standpoints. Our study highlights how these dimensions are influenced by traditional womanist studies; therefore, these methodological dimensions are derived from our main findings in chapters 2–5. To demonstrate the methodological and analytical use of these dimensions, we supplement our discussion with particular points of data from our study.

1) Storytelling

In line with previous research that focuses on womanist methods, a central theme in our interviews primarily focused on storytelling, or the ability and desire to share one's story. When asked if activism is part of her identity, 53-year-old activist Cinnamon from New York City responded,

> *No, I don't . . . I don't go around saying that I am an activist. I just basically [engage in activism] because it just comes natural to me as far as being an HIV [positive] African American woman. You know, I don't say that. I don't go around saying that I'm an activist for HIV; I just basically, you know, share. But I am an activist, but I don't, you know, it's not . . . I don't go around publicizing that I'm an activist. I just share my story. But I share basically with the women that are HIV, because they could identify with me, as well as me identifying with them as being HIV.*

Cinnamon "shared her story" and her personal experience; however, in her account, she described storytelling explicitly. This contrasts with 45-year-old Autumn, also from New York City, who shared her experiences confronting AIDS misinformation: "I am so grateful to [a local AIDS organization] because my daughter would not let me hold my only grandbaby because I'm HIV-positive and you know she came with me to [the local AIDS organization] and you know she now understands that you don't get [HIV] from holding." Autumn describes another instance of AIDS discrimination:

> *This is a true story . . . my landlord wanted my apartment because it was rent control and he threatened to tell all of the neighbors that I was living with HIV. I came to [local AIDS organization] and said that is so illegal I can't tell you how illegal that is. And so essentially the attorneys got to write a cease and desist order and get that person off my back.*

In both cases, Autumn shared two stories that detailed how AIDS has impacted her relationships with her daughter and her landlord. Thus, stories can be told both implicitly and explicitly. In line with most humanistic and social scientific methodologies that centralize womanism as their core epistemology, storytelling is the cornerstone for all of womanist literature and thought.

Thus, while womanism centers storytelling as part of its framework, story-telling is central to an empirical womanist methodology and measurement in womanist analysis.

2) Structurally Marginalized Identities and Community Structures

In chapter 2, we highlighted how notions of feminism conflate Black women's histories in health activism, nurturing, and caregiving within Black women's communities. After examining the literature, we found that the women in our sample were motivated by their immediate community structures. In order to conduct womanist research, we suggest that researchers examine how community structures impact structurally marginalized groups. To do so, our data offers two main dimensions of how womanist researchers could improve their methodological modes of inquiry: addressing interlocking structures and addressing cultural-historical conditions of behavior.

Interlocking Structures

Another dimension of expanding a womanist-based analysis is to highlight how interlocking structures impact how Black women and other structurally marginalized groups engage in health activism. For example, as mentioned in the second chapter, we present the following quote from Isabella, a 41-year-old women's program coordinator in Los Angeles:

> *Address the underlying issue, and the underlying issue is if you have a high unemployment and you have a high substance abuse and alcoholism, that puts people at risk. Meaning if you're unemployed, you're thinking about you might be depressed, and if you're depressed, the way that you cope with it—some people—is that they use alcohol or drugs. Then on top of that, if you have mass incarceration of a population, then for the women they're dealing with concurrent relationships. So, their main man is incarcerated, but they may feel that they need to have another relationship in order to get their needs met. So, I think by having those social injustices that's brought on, I think it will drive an epidemic in our community.*

Isabella describes how Black communities essentially have multiple concerns navigating AIDS, including mass incarceration, substance abuse, mental health concerns, and unemployment. In these concerns, Isabella highlights how Black individuals also navigate racial inequities along with multiple oppressive structures. While our respondents in chapter 2 demonstrate the need to examine these community structures, the data also demonstrates that, from a methodological perspective, womanist research should also examine how respondents navigate community structures. Based on Glenda's analysis that

AIDS "highlighted the unfairness, disparity, racism, [and] sexism . . . [as well as] psychosocial, economic, societal issues. . . . We've got to end all of those things so that we can end HIV/AIDS," understanding community structures and understanding individuals' experiences with interlocking inequities are important dimensions for womanist analysis.

Another dimension of examining community structures is to examine the historicity of structurally marginalized identities. In chapter 2, when some respondents explained the reasons why they understood themselves as activists, we contextualized these motivations of wanting to engage in community health activism as part of a cultural need to nurture. As Shay, a 56-year-old counselor and peer advocate for an AIDS service organization in rural South Carolina, explained in the second chapter, "Part of being an activist is being a spokesperson that speaks out and that believes in their cause and, and, going back again. I think I'm more stronger after that because I care. My whole thing is that I care about people." Shay describes how her caring nature empowers her to engage in activism and motivates her to care for other individuals. Thus, when engaging in a womanist analysis, it is important to highlight the historical and cultural context by which structurally marginalized communities engage in activism.

By identifying interlocking structures and cultural-historical conditions, womanist-based methodologies can examine a multifaceted approach that considers the historically and culturally specific conditions through which structurally marginalized individuals form their collective identities. Furthermore, womanist researchers can examine the confluence of an array of inequities that affect a particular group. They can also probe within these specific inequities in order to provide detail and nuance to a womanist analysis.

In addition to understanding how interlocking experiences impact structurally marginalized communities, researchers can understand how current and historical dimensions shape structurally marginalized groups and their behavior. For further examination, these methods can be combined to examine the historical and cultural impact of how these interlocking systems affect a structurally marginalized group.

3) Higher Power

In chapter 3, the respondents described how a belief in a higher power motivated their activism. As the 51-year-old founder of a New York City-based AIDS service organization working with formerly incarcerated women, Jasmine noted: "I'm a very spiritual person. I believe in my higher power. I understand the role of church or organized religion in my community. . . . I understand that the man standing in the pulpit is just a man and he is the messenger bringing the word of God and nothing more." While Jasmine acknowledges the importance of a higher power that guides her belief system, she also differentiates her belief system from a formal religious context.

Literature applying womanist methodologies suggests that religion influences respondents' experiences. However, it is important for womanist methodological frameworks to focus on the belief in one "higher power" (or spirituality), especially when examining Black women, as a key metric for conducting womanist research. This is especially relevant given that the women in our study reported that they veer away from the Black Church as their main cultural institution. When describing challenges to AIDS activism, 46-year-old New Orleans activist Lily explains that clergy often prevent women and LGBTQ+ people from gaining power: "Tons of challenges and resistance because there are a lot of folks who don't want women to have power. [They] don't want to have gay men to have power. They don't want the power basis of the church or the synagogue or mosque to be disrupted." Lily further argues that the main challenge to AIDS activism comes largely from clergy:

Clergy, heads of, you know, the religious dioceses, synagogue, and things. . . . [T]hen you have heads of the religion and [religious elected officials]. I think a lot of them have to do with being closeted themselves, not just about their sexual orientation, but their desires. [I'm] not saying they're all gays, but what do you enjoy when you're not allowing yourself to enjoy and the fact that so many have lied. It's like when a celebrity lied about, "I've been straight. I've been married. [But] 20 years later, knowing I have been really gay." It's the same thing. So, it's people with power like clergy like celebrity heads of company. They refuse to address the issues about HIV and AIDS because of their own internalized shame, stigma, whatever their issues are.

Here, this respondent describes how her experiences with Black churches were negatively impacted by homophobia and sexism. Clergy also maintain various forms of inequity that prevent AIDS activism. Thus, as shown in chapter 3, we suggest that future metrics focus on the notion of a "higher power," or spirituality, in order to examine how Black women and other structurally marginalized groups connect with divine forces while being inclusive of the notion of an Abrahamic God.

4) Embodied Actions

The relationship between structurally marginalized communities, interlocking experiences, religion, and spirituality are all imperative dimensions for womanist analysis. However, we highlight the notion that womanism can also expand on relationships between women of color's communities and the physical consequences of their community relationships.

In chapter 4, the respondents described how love and anger motivated their activism. In terms of love, our respondents described that it was love for their communities that enabled them to engage in activism. Thirty-one-year-old Tracy, who works in AIDS outreach and advocacy in Philadelphia, describes how love for her community members motivates her to continue to mobilize against AIDS. For example, Tracy explains,

> *I think with most AIDS activism work, if you've been infected, that's really what pushes a lot of people toward working with [AIDS]. And if you know someone who is infected, I think that is part of it. And then if you just have a concern for the overall, the people that are around you, if you, yourself, are involved in relationships and you're concerned with the men in your lives, the women in your lives, if you have little brothers, sisters, cousins, whatever, you feel that connection to teach others because you have young ones or people that you want to protect, I think that motivates people to get involved. But I think the majority of people, especially dealing with HIV and AIDS, the main thing that kind of motivates a lot of them is that they themselves have been infected, and then that pushes them to become involved.*

While Tracy explains that her community ties motivate her activism, others, like 51-year-old Jocelyn from New York City, maintained: "My friends were dying. . . . The first love of my life . . . his name is Max and he died of AIDS."

Thus, the women in our study act out of the love they have for community members and out of their positive community ties. While these women are driven by the love they have for their community members, they are also driven by anger. Ena, a 66-year-old Oakland-based activist and former sex worker, suggests,

> *Well with HIV specifically, was the fact that first they were scapegoating sex workers, so that got me involved with it, got me kind of angry and I knew that in order to make a difference I had to show my face because a lot of the women that I was working with were not African American. And to really make a difference, I felt like African Americans needed to have a voice, and lots of people, most people, don't want to talk about sex work if they have been involved in it. And so, being that my family and my friends and other people knew what my background was and didn't have a problem with it, I felt like I really needed to be out there.*

Here, Ena felt her community members were "scapegoated" as the source of HIV infection and their concerns were not validated. Similarly, Eulene, a 47-year-old New Yorker, who works in a public interest law firm, explains,

I think it starts with the personal. It has to. Maybe not has to, but it definitely starts with some kind of personal insult that things are a certain way. . . . There were people that I had the experience working around [she then names a local community activist]. She was a well-known obstetrician, but she became an activist around a host of issues because she was primarily serving Black women in Harlem and what she kept seeing unaddressed by other health care providers and by other social services, she started speaking out about it. She ended up becoming, you know, that's the danger too, that when we're really angry, we get written off as stringent and as, you know, kind of not able to be constructive, quote unquote. So, what motivates us, I think it's totally individual, but it's gotta have something to do, or at least in my experience, and with the people I've worked with and the women I've worked with, it's just an unwillingness to accept a kind of that's just the way it is.

Eulene recalled how health providers ignored her community's struggles. She also reported an inability to accept health inequities as the status quo. These factors motivated her activism. Finally, Virginia, a 50-year-old AIDS educator who lives and works in Philadelphia, describes how feelings of solidarity influence why she mobilizes against AIDS:

The primary reason why I got involved is I am, actually, I am a woman living with the virus. The second primary reason is because I have a sister who lost her fight to an AIDS-related illness back in the early '80s. So, you know, losing her and the way she, you know, the services that were not there for her just inspired me to make sure that . . . that I would be there at the table to make sure that when it comes to services, that what people need for HIV and AIDS, that they receive.

Thus, in addition to living with HIV, feelings of solidarity and the loss of her sister inspire Virginia's activism work. As such, this research has shown that emotions such as love, anger, and feelings of solidarity affect how Black women engage in activism.

As explored in chapter 4, emotions were key to developing an emotionally based practice that centered around the relationships these women have with their communities. We mainly find that these emotions are driven by the respondents' lived experiences, and the respondents pragmatically act in response to inequity. Thus, given that these emotions have biological, psychological, and social components, they are *viscerally embodied* in that these emotions are both felt and experienced within a social context.

Black women's connection between themselves and their communities generates visceral experiences of love and anger. These community ties elicit a physiological connection between Black women's bodies and their communities. As a result of the physiological response to how Black women understand AIDS activism through their emotions, we argue that Black women *embody* their experiences.

A womanist methodological framework can highlight how structurally marginalized communities embody both the experience and resistance of social inequities. In the examples above, the respondents resist health inequities by continuing to mobilize against AIDS. The women in our study continue to mobilize against AIDS out of the love they have for their community members. At the same time, these feelings of loss are driven by inequity. By experiencing love and anger, Black women embody these feelings in structurally marginalized contexts, and, therefore, womanist methodological frameworks should affirm emotions as an analytical focal point.

5) Knowledge Transmission

As mentioned above, knowledge transmission (via storytelling methods) is a defining feature of womanism. With storytelling being at the forefront of womanist epistemology and methodology, womanism emphasizes knowledge transmission, including the accessibility to acquire this knowledge. For example, Crystal, a board member at an AIDS organization in the South, suggests,

> *My agency was founded on prevention. . . . Our anchor service is testing—knowing your status, making it accessible, available; reducing stigma so that people will get tested and know their status; integrating it into normalizing it; routine. And educating about what you do now and what you should do in the future if you don't want to be infected. And within that, we end up identifying and serving people living with HIV.*

In her suggestion, Crystal explains that "knowing" one's HIV status and "educating" others to prevent HIV transmission are imperative in community relations. As a result, the women in our study acknowledge that AIDS information itself and the transmission of AIDS information are important to community survival. However, in addition to storytelling, we posit the notion that there are two main "vectors" of how knowledge transmission occurs: cultural authorities and institutions.

Cultural Authorities

In terms of cultural authorities, the respondents explained the relationship between Black Church officials and the spread of AIDS information. For example, Shay explains the relationship with clergy and officials by noting:

> *We need more people to get involved in it. And I'm talking about, like, outside resources such as, like, our ministers and people of that nature, where people*

tend to, like, listen to. They talk about other illnesses, but a lot of them don't talk about the HIV virus. Now, I have been to churches that have talked about it, that, like, the church I was going in New York, we had groups of certain nights, you know. I was really into getting involved in the HIV project.

In HIV prevention efforts, she mentions that she needed more involvement from religious institutions because parishioners listen to church authorities, such as ministers. While highlighting the importance of sharing and storytelling, Shay suggests that authority figures are not sharing AIDS information and AIDS-related stories. Thus, authority figures with significant cultural capital are very important from a womanist perspective because their ability to share stories can strongly impact their communities.

Culturally Relevant Institutions

Authorities with cultural capital also affect knowledge transmission, especially when access to these institutional resources affects HIV prevention. Fifty-six-year-old AIDS advocate and educator Beatrice highlights how access to medical institutions is critical to HIV prevention within Black communities:

Well, I think it's, first of all, actually letting Black people know the extent of the disease within the community, right? That would be the first step, I think, and assisting them in how to maneuver the particular systems that are in place to help them because people have no idea. I even look at even when you go to any sort of hospital or any sort of institution, it's how do you maneuver in that institution? How do you know, get to see the doctor, see the nurse, see the case manager without actually going bonkers about how to figure it out, right? So, it's about access; I think it's access to education, I think it's access to health care, I think it's access to housing, it's drugs, child care, all sort of things.

Essentially, Beatrice expresses several concerns: the lack of knowledge of AIDS information within Black communities, the lack of knowledge of how HIV is spread, and the lack of knowledge about accessing AIDS treatment. Thus, another component of knowledge transmission is the ability to navigate health institutions, which would help promote longevity and health within Black communities.

Finally, the last dimension of knowledge transmission is the ability for communities to develop culturally relevant institutions. As discussed in chapter 5, in explaining the need for sexual education, Tracy says,

If as a society we're making any changes towards what occurs, you need to lay that seed. And I think if you have that education in the schools, people have a better idea of what's going on with their bodies, how what they do will have

an impact on their body. Then as a society, as they're older. They'll have the tools to make the decisions from there. . . . But I don't even think we're giving anyone the proper tools to make the better decisions. It's just kind of, "We'll give a class for two days in eighth grade," but something may have already occurred by then, so the tools aren't really there or in place. So as a society, I think it really started with providing that proper education for them but, even that's difficult, because if you look at the schools now and everything, they're cutting, then that'll go, that'll open another door of issues. So, I mean, I think it's an idealistic approach to it, but I think it's important.

Tracy discusses the importance of the expansion of sex education within the public-school system and its vulnerability to budget cuts. In this context, Tracy argues that institutions that deploy AIDS information are necessary because this information affects how individuals within her community regulate their sexual behavior. Tracy suggests that if those in her community receive sexual education, they will "have a better idea of what's going on with their bodies [and] have tools to make the decisions." Thus, womanist methodological frameworks can account for the importance of culturally relevant institutions.

In sum, womanist methodological frameworks can evolve and incorporate the need to focus on cultural authorities, the ability to navigate institutions, and finally, the ability to have institutions serve the interests of structurally marginalized communities. Thus, a womanist methodological framework considers these dimensions of knowledge transmission and storytelling.

TOWARD AN EMBODIED WOMANIST METHOD

Based on our results, we propose to expand womanist methodologies through what we call the "embodied womanist methodology." This methodology expands womanist methodologies by addressing several key components: cultural and historical community relations, proximity to interlocking inequities, religion/spiritual dichotomy, physical embodiments, and cultural and epistemological authority. This methodology has the following main assumptions:

1. Storytelling as the validation for experience.

   A defining feature in womanist analysis is the notion that storytelling validates how Black women and those from other structurally marginalized communities develop knowledge unique to their experiences. However, while this is the foundation through which womanist analyses are conducted, storytelling can indeed be nuanced for further analytical and explanatory power.

2. The researcher validates that any structurally marginalized identity exists in relation to historical and cultural conditions.

   At present, womanist literature contextualizes Black women's experiences in a time-specific locale, and it attempts to address cultural variation within strands of Africana womanist thought. This particular addition can help researchers address the socio-historical conditions of Black women and the experiences of other structurally marginalized women.

3. The researcher assesses the proximity between the structurally marginalized identity and its relationship to interlocking modes of inequity.

   Womanist literature focuses on three main dimensions: storytelling, empowerment, and spirituality. However, when examining inequity, womanist approaches affirm the cultural facets of Black women's experiences, but do not focus on how different modes of inequity affect Black women's connection to their community. Through focusing on the proximity of structurally marginalized identities and focusing on how individuals navigate systems of inequity, researchers can examine the impact of social inequities on the experiences of structurally marginalized groups. Researchers can also pinpoint specific factors that affect how structurally marginalized people navigate social inequity and highlight spaces and sources for resiliency.

4. The researcher acknowledges the notion of the "higher power," its relationship to religion and religious institutions, and its motivation toward action.

   Our respondents note that not only are there differences between religiosity and spirituality, but, also, their sense of spirituality is derived from their experiences with religion. Thus, womanist researchers must also focus their analysis on the relationship between "higher powers" and understandings of "God." Furthermore, researchers should also demonstrate the factors that affect the disjuncture between spirituality and religion.

5. The researcher affirms how physical phenomena relate to the structurally marginalized community's experience.

   Our data specifically examined how emotions motivate Black women into mobilizing against AIDS. However, emotions have both physiological and social components. Thus, researchers can also examine how bodies are affected by structurally marginalized experiences, community bonds, and connectedness.

6. The researcher notes appropriate vectors of cultural significance and knowledge authorities.

From this method, structurally marginalized identities are contextualized within a framework of community relations, social relations, and bodily relations. Thus, the method then is able to expand on womanist principles while also contributing to a larger methodology of Black feminist research.

By applying embodied womanist methodologies, the researcher is able to treat race and gender as a collective experience rather than an experience that activates at different intervals at various times. This methodology enables the researcher to develop a sense of cultural and social historicity and to simultaneously address how individuals from structurally marginalized groups navigate interlocking structures of inequity. Furthermore, this womanist methodology is able to affirm the spiritualities of structurally marginalized individuals, as with previous literature in womanist methods, but also able to derive how religion and religious institutions affect the formation of spirituality. Furthermore, this perspective enables the researcher to be aware of the relationship between the body and community connectedness. Finally, the embodied womanist perspective enables the researcher to examine major vectors of culturally specific authorities and institutions that shape community involvement.

EMBODIED WOMANIST RESEARCH BENEFITS AND LIMITATIONS

In their totality, embodied womanist principles can benefit researchers by expanding studies of inequity, especially because the methodology examines particular cultural components and historical conditions that influence how structurally marginalized identities resist interlocking modes of inequity. These principles can highlight distinctions and similarities of how constructs, such as religion and spirituality, explain behavior. The methodology can also examine the visceral impact of community bonds and the impact on various structural outcomes. Additionally, researchers can address how "storytelling" functions by identifying modes of knowledge transmission. Finally, the main principles of embodied womanist methodology can influence quantitative and qualitative research principles.

In terms of quantitative and survey-based research, we argue that these dimensions can further be explored in terms of survey construction and index construction. These metrics can be validated through reliability and validity checks, or they can be tested empirically via ordinary least squares, logistic regression, or hierarchical modeling techniques.

In addition, with qualitative research, our principles can guide researchers to map general areas of how to study structurally marginalized experiences. For example, a researcher can focus on one of the five dimensions that we identify by developing a research methodology that incorporates one of the embodied womanist principles. By doing so, the researchers could incorporate storytelling in addition to developing other metrics that focus on spirituality. Likewise, a researcher could draft a "map" (a physical representation of specific ideas) that triangulates each embodied womanist principle with one another within given populations. This would be done in an effort to examine how structurally marginalized experiences occur within a particular community by incorporating a number of research methods including interview, narrative analysis, ethnography, or other critical discourse methodologies. Indeed, by applying embodied womanist principles as a "mapping exercise," a researcher could possibly create a historically and culturally nuanced "picture" of the experiences of those from structurally marginalized communities.

While there are benefits to applying embodied womanist principles in social research, there are also limitations. For example, our methodology is based on the experiences of Black women. Given that womanism encompasses experiences of structurally marginalized communities—without respect to race, gender, or other structurally marginalized statuses—future methodological advancements can also consider other women of color as well as other aspects of structurally marginalized experiences. Furthermore, this methodological perspective suggests that the research occurs outside of a neocolonial context; thus, for future iterations of this methodology, we argue that colonialism should be factored into subsequent epistemological and methodological advancements. Critical race and feminist perspectives (and even intersectionality to some extent) analyze dominant identities in addition to structurally marginalized identities. In contrast, womanism is a perspective that focuses almost exclusively on the experiences of structurally marginalized groups. Thus, while we lay the groundwork for future analyses in examining marginalization, we suggest that future womanist perspectives can develop methodologies that examine the experiences of dominant perspectives.

Furthermore, while we posit dimensions of womanist research and describe potential applications in social research, our goal is to simply provide a guide on how to apply these principles quantitatively and qualitatively. We do not detail precise research designs that have applied this methodological framework; we simply provide suggestions.

ADDRESSING GAPS IN METHODOLOGICAL LITERATURE

Intersectional research methods primarily focus on developing identity-based arguments that demonstrate the unique conditions that individual groups experience. Usually, these identity-based arguments focus squarely on the identities they seek to study, or they offer a comparative approach. Additionally, intersectionality-based methods are used to examine variations within a particular group. However, they do not consider the formation of intra-community ties, experiences with emotions, specific development of social institutions, or a historical analysis of these structures. In addition, intersectional literature and methods would argue that inhabiting a religious or spiritual identity depends on multiple factors and affects one's outcome. However, the main limitation with intersectional literature is that it suggests that religion and spirituality are clear units of analysis that yield particular outcomes.

Womanism, in contrast, highlights community ties and relations, the importance of spirituality, social change, lived experiences, and storytelling. As womanism is a stronger epistemological and methodological framework compared to intersectional frameworks, our theories expand upon womanist methodologies.

We argue that our data addresses both cultural and historical dimensions to the study of structurally marginalized communities as they interact with interlocking structures of inequity, whereas at present, womanist empirical research does not provide cultural and historical variation. Furthermore, womanist methodologies emphasize spirituality; however, they do not differentiate religion from spirituality, examine the derivation of spirituality from religion, nor describe religion and spirituality's relationship to other forms of social inequity.

While womanist research focuses on lived experiences, it does not focus on how these experiences are embodied. We find that Black women's emotions help motivate their social organizing, as such, we suggest that researchers focus on how the experiences of Black women and other structurally marginalized women are embodied.

Finally, womanism places an emphasis on community storytelling; however, womanist methodological approaches do not specify how community institutions address knowledge production within structurally marginalized communities. Our data identifies how cultural authorities, institutions dominated by nonstructurally marginalized communities, and institutions created by structurally marginalized communities affect knowledge transmission. Thus, by positing the notion of an embodied womanist methodology, we suggest directions for future empirical research that adopts a womanist framework.

CONCLUSION

In the context of how Black communities are impacted by AIDS, our manuscript addresses the question: What encourages AIDS activism among Black women? To answer this question, we apply a womanist framework because womanism addresses how structurally marginalized communities find empowerment, incorporate spirituality, emphasize the community bond, and enact social change.

After interviewing 36 Black women AIDS activists, we found that these women engage in activism to affirm how intersecting inequities affect their communities, and they do not privilege their experiences with sexism over other inequities that affect Black communities. We also found that our respondents maintained a sense of spirituality once they transitioned away from their religious upbringings. Furthermore, we described how our respondents were motivated by emotions because of their community ties. Finally, we found that the suggestions for social change that were posited by the women in our study can help provide specific direction on community-specific programs and approaches to addressing AIDS in their communities.

Study findings not only address limitations within existing Black feminist studies on AIDS, but these findings also expand on how womanism applies to AIDS activism, empirical Black feminist research, health policy, and non-profit activism. In addition to making contributions to epistemological frameworks in Black feminism, intersectionality, and womanism, we also contribute to methodological frameworks within Black feminism, intersectionality, and womanism specifically by being able to address how these Black feminist perspectives engage in empirical research.

In this section, we review intersectionality as it relates to intersectional methodological practice and womanist theory as it relates to womanist methodological practice. We also discuss these frameworks and their limitations. In terms of intersectionality as a framework, intersectionality is mainly an analytic perspective that enables researchers to parse out specific identities as they relate to specific outcomes (health or other outcomes). On the other hand, while womanist thought addresses the limitations of intersectionality, its main concepts can be further expanded in order to promote analytic rigor.

Therefore, in order to expand on womanist research methodologies, we highlight key findings from our data set and expand upon their potential to contribute to womanist research methodology. The first main finding is that storytelling is central to womanist analyses. Throughout our analysis, we privilege our respondents' stories, but we also identify that there are two main ways to identify storytelling whether it be explicit—"I shared my story . . ."— or implicit—recounting an experience to demonstrate a concept. Through identifying storytelling as the main mode of womanist analyses, we align ourselves with traditional womanist thought and its methodologies. We then expand traditional womanist methodologies by identifying four other dimensions of womanist thought.

First, we highlight how womanist methodologies should identify how interlocking modes of inequity affect the experiences of Black women and other structurally marginalized communities. By identifying interlocking inequities, womanist analyses can highlight how Black women and other structurally marginalized women experience inequities and also resist inequities. Additionally, researchers can pinpoint culturally and historically specific factors that affect Black women's experiences, and they can determine that these experiences can be traced along various historical and cultural lineages. Thus, researchers can consider cultural context and the historicity of their arguments by applying this research strategy.

Secondly, we describe how womanist methodologies highlight the relationship between spirituality and structurally marginalized identities. While our work aligns with traditional research on womanist thought, our findings demonstrate how those from structurally marginalized identities incorporate spirituality as a key aspect of their identity. Previous womanist analyses have applied hermeneutical methodologies to study religion's impact on the development of identities, but we suggest that researchers should trace how Black women and other structurally marginalized groups understand their spiritualities in relation to, but separate from, religion.

Next, we suggest that womanist analyses should also consider how experiences are viscerally embodied. After finding that our respondents' community ties motivate their activism, we argue these emotions (grounded in biological and physiological processes) impact how Black women are physically affected by these ties. Thus, womanist methodologies should also include an examination between structurally marginalized communities, their emotions, and their community ties.

Finally, we argue that womanist analyses could also focus on institutions that produce culturally specific sites of knowledge transmittal. We find that cultural institutions and authorities produce information that enables individuals to access healthcare, and that these factors might influence how communities navigate social concerns. Likewise, from a womanist perspective, it is important to assess how structurally marginalized individuals navigate spaces that are not historically amenable to their experiences. We find that womanist methodologies can also account for how structurally marginalized experiences produce their own institutions in order to deploy culturally sensitive information for community members.

From these six main dimensions of how our data shapes womanist episte-mology, we then posit a specific methodology of how to engage womanist theory from a methodological perspective called "embodied womanist meth-odology." Embodied womanist methodology has six main principles: story-telling, validating cultural and historical identities, interlocking structures, spirituality, embodied actions, and knowledge transmission. By identifying these main principles, we create expanded dimensions of womanism to help empirical researchers focus on one or multiple parts of womanist analyses.

Central to womanist research, the first principle of storytelling is central to womanist analysis, methodologies, and epistemology. The second principle validates Black women's cultural and historical circumstances. The third principle involves identifying interlocking modes of inequity and their prox-imity to structurally marginalized experiences. The fourth principle involves recognizing the relationship between religion, spirituality, and structurally marginalized experiences. The fifth principle involves examining the rela-tionship between structurally marginalized experiences and embodiment. The last principle involves examining how structurally marginalized communities frame and transmit information as culturally palatable.

The main advantages of the embodied womanist perspective is that this perspective accounts for the historicity of structurally marginalized experi-ences, community-specific patterns in relation to interlocking structures, nu-ances of religion and spirituality, lived experiences and community ties, and community-specific modes of knowledge dissemination. Focusing on these five main dimensions of experiences, researchers can understand inequity by gauging how communities relate to intersecting experiences and oppressions.

Given these principles, embodied womanism is a methodological per-spective that enables researchers to document different aspects of womanist analysis and to maintain womanism's focus on storytelling, empowerment, and spirituality. Embodied womanism seeks to flesh out specific analyti-cal dimensions in order to highlight womanism's epistemological strengths within an empirical research context.

In addition to storytelling, we also account for historical and cultural nature of experiences; interaction with interlocking systems of power; gradations of religiosity and spirituality; experiences with emotions; and knowledge formations within structurally marginalized communities. Likewise, our syn-thesis primarily focuses on the experiences of Black women. Even though womanism has focused primarily on African, Afro-Caribbean, and African-American perspectives of experiences, womanism has been applied to other women of color communities, such as Latinx and Asian communities.

Appendix B

The Activists and Their Stories

In this book, we describe how Black women AIDS activists mobilize against AIDS in their communities, and we find that womanist frameworks best explain how Black women are motivated to lead their communities against AIDS. We argue that community consciousness, religion/spirituality, emotions, and the women's suggestions for change play a role in addressing critical processes and explanations of Black women's mobilization against AIDS. First, respondents described how a need to protect their communities fueled their activism. They also explained how other factors outside of gender inequity, such as racial and economic inequities, affected their communities. Next, the respondents explained that they distinguished between religiosity and spirituality. Their experiences with religiosity were affected by their experiences working in and worshipping in Black churches. They also highlighted how their experiences with homophobia and sexism stymied their activism work. The respondents felt love for their communities, pain for their lost loved ones, and solidarity with others. Finally, the respondents highlighted suggestions for social change.

While there were patterns in how respondents engaged in AIDS activism, we also want to highlight each respondent's story. In line with womanist frameworks that emphasize storytelling, we can learn more about these activists by hearing their stories and learning about their experiences mobilizing against AIDS in their communities. Below we provide a brief description of each activist in our study, including their age, sexuality, where they live, the type of activism in which they are engaged, and how they understand their work.

ALYSSA, EARLY THIRTIES, HETEROSEXUAL, BROOKLYN, NY—COMMUNITY ACTIVIST

Alyssa comes from a family of West Indian immigrants, and she grew up in a working-class community. Alyssa's family valued education. Her grandparents, especially her grandmother, motivated her studies and encouraged her to pursue higher education after high school. Alyssa thrived as a psychology major at her East Coast university, gained ample enrichment opportunities and support, and earned her bachelor's degree. Later, as a social services practitioner and a Christian, Alyssa found that her religious beliefs taught her the compassion and patience she needed to succeed in her career. She was in a relationship at the time of the interview.

In her AIDS activism work, Alyssa serves as an AIDS advocate and provides sex education and paraphernalia for West-Indian and Latinx women and encourages HIV testing in undocumented and immigrant communities. Working with teenagers and the elderly, Alyssa encourages these individuals to practice safer sex. She also teaches HIV-positive individuals about the importance of properly taking medications. Professionally, Alyssa provides education, resources, and support to HIV-positive patients in her program. In addition, she has a number of managerial responsibilities, such as supervising staff and budgeting.

The core of Alyssa's activism is self-advocacy, and she advocates for women's sexual autonomy and their ability to negotiate condom use. For example, she finds that some women resist condoms because they do not know about safer sex practices or they are afraid of being labeled as sexually promiscuous. Alyssa noted that in both her work in the U.S. and Haiti, some women also fear discussing their sexual health with their doctor while others believe that they are in monogamous relationships but later find out their partner is unfaithful. To address these challenges, Alyssa believes that if women can advocate for themselves, regardless of country, they can better protect themselves from HIV.

AUTUMN, 45, QUEER, NEW YORK CITY, NY—EXECUTIVE DIRECTOR OF HEALTH SERVICE ORGANIZATION

Autumn was raised in a deeply religious and politically engaged matriarchal family in New York City. Later, Autumn would have a daughter. Autumn recounted her early experiences, when she began her activism as a teenager when she donated to a fund to end mass incarceration. She later focused on

AIDS activism when a female friend who was HIV-positive had difficulty accessing treatment because most services were dedicated to men.

Autumn's serves as an Executive Director of an AIDS organization that targets primarily Black communities by providing mental health services, AIDS education, and resources (e.g., career consulting and legal services). Having earned her doctorate, she worked as a licensed psychologist in government and nonprofit sectors. In particular, she worked with one nonprofit that targeted Black lesbians.

Activism is a core part of Autumn's identity. However, her primary challenge is funding. Autumn suggests that activists need to be able to better utilize their resources when they meet multiple demands. For example, Autumn describes the opportunity costs when developing a campaign where activists must choose between funding more testing or outreach. To combat these issues, Autumn holds major fundraising events, such as an AIDS Walk.

BETTY, 53, HETEROSEXUAL, BALTIMORE, MD— AIDS MOTIVATIONAL SPEAKER AND WOMEN'S HEALTH ADVOCATE

Betty was born in the Bronx. Upon her mother's death, Betty's grandparents raised her. Although she now identifies as spiritual instead of religious, she grew up in a traditionally religious home and was raised Protestant. She also earned an associate's degree. She now is married with four adult children and several grandchildren. As someone who is HIV-positive, Betty became involved in AIDS work as she first simply wanted to learn about what to expect as a person living with HIV. She soon found herself fielding HIV-related questions from community members and advocating for those with AIDS.

As both part of her paid and volunteer AIDS advocacy work, Betty teaches her community members about safer sex behaviors and condom use, and, also, she helps women secure housing, food, and navigate doctor's appointments. She is a public speaker who shares her lived experiences with others and serves as a speaker and advocate. Betty works at an AIDS organization that provided AIDS education to community members. Once these individuals received a certain amount of education and training, they were then charged with providing AIDS education to other community members—a "train the trainer" model.

The primary philosophy in Betty's activism is to focus on education and "Just to keep the people aware. Every day, keep them aware." Through education, Betty believes that her clients can understand how their sexual choices impact the spread of HIV. Her ability to relay information has been effective, especially since others have told her, "The condoms that you gave me and showed me how to use, I use them now." However, Betty encounters a number of challenges in her work, primarily funding. She believes that a lack of funding can curtail these efforts because, for example, AIDS education and support groups often fail because, as she explained, they cannot afford to maintain their physical location. This is especially problematic in underserved areas where individuals drive long distances to get access to these support groups and programs.

BEATRICE, 56, HETEROSEXUAL, NEW YORK CITY, NY— COMMUNITY ACTIVIST AND AIDS EDUCATOR

Beatrice was raised in Brooklyn. Her mother was from the South and her father was from Trinidad. Her mother worked as a respiratory therapist and nurse, while her father, a former Marine, owned a business. Her mother, grandmother, and great-grandmother were politically active. Her mother was active in community service, while her grandmother and great-grandmother founded a church in their local community. Beatrice completed college and went on to earn her doctorate. She is married without children. Seeing activism as important, Beatrice became motivated to engage in AIDS activism work to protect, as she described, "Black women, infants, and children" from the impact of AIDS.

Beatrice's activism focuses on education and community advocacy. Beatrice develops relationships with Congressional officials and state and local legislatures, providing these groups with AIDS information, including disease rates in her local community, and leads her community's advocacy and support.

Beatrice notes a number of accomplishments that resulted from her activism work that she finds inspirational; for example, in addition to the passage of certain legislation that supports those with HIV, Beatrice finds that many of her community members report that they feel much more comfortable and empowered when they openly discuss sex and sexuality and advocate for their own sexual health. The primary challenge she faces in her work is AIDS stigma. She maintains that since the government did not target Black communities in initial AIDS education campaigns, it is hard for many in Black communities to take the illness seriously and engage in safer sex practices.

BRIANNA, 58, HETEROSEXUAL, ORANGEBURG, SC— COMMUNITY ACTIVIST AND AIDS MOTIVATIONAL SPEAKER

Brianna grew up in a larger family on the Lower East Side of Manhattan. Brianna eventually earned her bachelor's degree and surpassed her family members in terms of her education. Her mother had some college education and worked as a nursery school teacher, and her father worked without a formal education. At the time of the interview, Brianna was married with children. After her eldest brother died of AIDS, Brianna relocated to South Carolina and began her involvement in AIDS ministry. Soon after, Brianna received an HIV-positive diagnosis herself, and coped with her illness through support groups. She then began to lobby Congress to expand services for HIV-positive communities during the AIDS epidemic's onset.

Brianna is a community activist and motivational speaker who largely works with HIV-positive individuals. As an activist, she develops support groups, and she helps individuals navigate their interactions with their medical providers. She also speaks on Ryan White Part D, a program that focuses on HIV-positive women and children. Brianna was previously unemployed but she founded two organizations, and volunteers as a program coordinator.

The core of Brianna's activism focuses on ending the criminalization of HIV. Brianna served jail time because of drug use and abuse. Since her time in jail, Brianna notes several hardships, including unemployment. She currently works to raise awareness about and end HIV criminalization laws. However, Brianna notes the stigma associated with addressing these laws.

CINNAMON, 53, HETEROSEXUAL, NEW YORK CITY, NY— AIDS HOUSING AND TREATMENT ACTIVIST

Cinnamon grew up in Harlem. Her mother was a single parent, but she also remained in contact with her father. Her parents sold drugs to support the family. Though she attempted to abstain from drug use, she engaged in substance abuse. She dropped out of high school, ran away from home, and became pregnant. She then returned home to have her daughter, stopped using drugs, and checked into a rehabilitation program. This program provided the training she needed to eventually become employed. Cinnamon supports others as they combat AIDS and began her activist career as someone who was HIV-positive herself. At the time of the interview, Cinnamon was in a relationship.

Cinnamon volunteers with multiple AIDS organizations and with a large AIDS activist group on the East Coast as a peer educator. In her role, she provides information about HIV programs and targets primarily women and men with HIV. In her activism, she encounters several challenges, especially when "Some people don't want to know. Some people don't want to be tested, scared to be tested, scared that they are positive and, and think that what they don't know won't hurt them—which, that is just totally crazy, I believe." Her activism is unpaid—she was unemployed at the time of the interview—she lives on Social Security and Disability.

Cinnamon engages in activism because she lives with HIV and she empathizes with individuals who also have the virus. Cinnamon suggests that activists educate other individuals about the impact the virus has on the body and how to effectively prevent and treat HIV infection. Specifically, she recounts how taking particular mediations did not help her manage her HIV, and that those medications had a deleterious effect on her body. Thus, she uses her own experiences with HIV in order to provide education to others. When asked about her successes, Cinnamon maintains that, "my successes are successfully living with [HIV] for 24 years. You know, that's a success because a lot of people have died."

CRYSTAL, AGE NOT DISCLOSED, HETEROSEXUAL, SOUTH CAROLINA—AIDS EDUCATOR AND ADVOCATE FOR RESEARCH

Born and raised in Upstate New York, Crystal sees herself as someone who has received a divine "calling" for work in AIDS community service. Crystal was inspired by her father, who rose through the ranks to become a public health executive in their local community, and she recalled how growing up she remembered him crying in the evenings after work as as he struggled to support his community and help others. Crystal never gets tired from activism because she sees her work's impact on others. She also has some college experience. Crystal is married with one child and has a grandchild. She is also deeply religious and works as an usher in her church. Believing that she's doing God's will, Crystal feels that her religious beliefs provide her with a sense of stability and support that helps guide her activism work.

Crystal engages in both paid and unpaid AIDS advocacy work and is a statewide chair for an AIDS nonprofit. In conjunction with focusing on research and serving on multiple boards, Crystal works with a variety of groups to lobby for more AIDS education resources and support to groups ranging from members of Congress, college students, and LGBTQ+ communities.

Additionally, she frequently presents and speaks at conferences, churches, and other institutions. Given that she has a doctorate and trained as a sexual health educator, Crystal taught a research-based sexual education program in her community.

Maintaining that she defines herself through her AIDS advocacy work, the primary goal of Crystal's activism is to provide AIDS education and resources to at-risk groups. However, she faces several challenges in her work. In addition to accessing and competing for the scarce AIDS funding available, Crystal describes how homophobia in Black communities has been a particularly difficult challenge to overcome as many heterosexuals do not see their own susceptibly to HIV infection. Overall, she believes that the government does very little to address the structural barriers that help cause increased rates of HIV in Black communities.

DANA, 59, HETEROSEXUAL, PHILADELPHIA, PA—WOMEN AND LGBTQ+ RIGHTS ACTIVIST AND AIDS EDUCATOR

Dana's mother and great-grandmother played a particularly important role in Dana's upbringing. Her grandmother was a pastor. But, at seventeen, Dana converted to Islam. In her twenties, she became a mother and parented three children. Dana also had some college experience. Dana is a Sunday school teacher who has several grandchildren and one great-grandchild. At the time of the interview, Dana was married.

Dana is a community advocate that primarily works with women, LGBTQ+ individuals, and communities of color because she served on boards, chaired committees, and founded several organizations. As an activist, she conducts basic training, collects signatures for petitions, and engages in "direct action." Dana works full time in the nonprofit sector and is fulfilled in her role as an HIV tester, where she was able to comfort newly diagnosed HIV-positive clients.

The core of Dana's activism is to improve the quality of life of other individuals. However, Dana finds that her activism can have limits. While Dana empowers others by showing them that they can make a difference in their communities, when these individuals begin to excel in activism, they are often offered careers in place of their activism. This can be disruptive because when these individuals will no longer have time to contribute to mobilizing others, this can have a detrimental impact on sustained leadership and continuity. Another challenge to her activism is illiteracy. Dana believes it's also important to "push more for adult education" because she finds "illiteracy" prevents AIDS education and overall health literacy.

DOROTHY, 50, QUEER, OAKLAND, CA—
COMMUNITY ACTIVIST

Dorothy identifies herself as an activist because she is, as she explains, "the type of individual that will stand up for . . . all the right things." A single parent, Dorothy always felt empowered by the women in her family, especially her mom and her sister. Dorothy began her activism when she learned about her own HIV-positive status. For a brief time, Dorothy lived in denial about her illness. However, she learned more about her illness through activism and relayed AIDS information, such as HIV's transmission, to her family members. Being educated about HIV helps Dorothy navigate her diagnosis and enables her family members to destigmatize the illness.

As a community advocate, Dorothy provides underprivileged, HIV-positive and AIDS patients with emotional support and medical and social work access. For example, Dorothy helps homeless women become financially stable. She also lobbies Congress for favorable AIDS legislation. However, her organization was experiencing cuts to funding, and this limits her ability to engage in activism.

Though she did not finish high school, Dorothy stresses the importance of education and believes, "There's not enough education going on." She ultimately wants to address how AIDS misinformation drives the AIDS epidemic in the United States. To curb the spread of misinformation, Dorothy encounters several challenges. She believes that AIDS stigma prevents younger generations from talking about the virus and spreading information about AIDS. She also wants individuals to be comfortable talking about condom use. Dorothy believes that some individuals need to know that they should not drink alcohol or do drugs before they have sex as it reduces their inhibitions and increases sexual risk-taking behaviors. AIDS information should also be inclusive of trans women's experiences. Finally, to address misinformation in heterosexual male communities, Dorothy believes that openly gay and bisexual men should educate heterosexual men about HIV risk-taking behaviors as they often know more than their heterosexual counterparts about HIV infection.

ESTELLE, 43, HETEROSEXUAL, NORTH CAROLINA—
COMMUNITY ACTIVIST AND AIDS EDUCATOR

Estelle believed she had a conventionally middle-class upbringing, where she participated in Girl Scouts, gymnastics, and music and she lived a sheltered lifestyle. Her mother worked for the government and was a secretary for her church. However, her life changed when she realized her father sold drugs.

She graduated from high school but also abused substances herself and soon tested positive for HIV. After her diagnosis, a clergy member who worked in an AIDS ministry inspired her to start a nonprofit. Eventually, she married and had two children.

Estelle engages in both community activism and AIDS education targeting primarily Black communities and gay and bisexual men. She is employed as a medical case manager and an HIV tester. She also works to educate lawmakers about AIDS-related issues, runs support groups, and provides AIDS and safer sex education.

Estelle's primary goals are to increase community awareness about AIDS, to reduce AIDS stigma, and to "continue to live." However, according to Estelle, denial and ignorance exacerbate the AIDS crisis in the United States. In her experience, structurally marginalized people are labeled as the "other," and, by labeling others, people fail to recognize their own susceptibility to HIV. Estelle believes that activists need more financial resources to continue to work, but this work is often "mind-numbing" and exhausting. Additionally, she believes churches are not really receptive to her messaging. Finally, she argues that those in more rural communities often have difficulty receiving access to services and treatment.

ENA, 66, QUEER, OAKLAND, CA—AIDS EDUCATOR AND SEX WORKER'S RIGHTS ACTIVIST

Ena was born in San Francisco and was raised alongside her seven siblings by her mother, who was a homemaker, and her father, who worked in a warehouse. Later, she went to college, but did not graduate. Ena is not married but has been in a relationship with a woman for almost 20 years and has two adult children. She was raised a Jehovah's Witness, but later converted to the Church of Religion and Science. Spiritualty plays a major part in Ena's life as it motivates her to overcome obstacles.

Ena is the founder and executive of a nonprofit that advocates for sex worker's rights, specifically targeting Black communities, other women of color, and sex workers. The primary goal of Ena's activism work is to ensure that sex workers and other structurally marginalized groups receive access to HIV prevention funding and services. To do so, she lobbies Congress and engages other political actors. She says, "We've done marches, we've done sit-ins, we've went to the Board of Supervisors, we've done lots of meetings. But probably the most effective thing, I think, is lobbying." She also works to dispel misconceptions about sex work, including that sex workers abuse illicit substances and/or are forced into sex work.

Working in community activism since around 1981, Ena first became interested in advocacy when, as a research participant in a sex worker study, she noticed that many of the sex workers in the study were not receiving accurate information regarding safer sex education and resources. She believed that the stigma associated with sex work negatively affected sex workers and dedicated her life to working to reduce stigmas facing sex workers, provide treatment for substance abuse, and provide safer sex education. However, Ena finds the stigmas associated with sex work to be the greatest challenge to her advocacy efforts.

GLENDA, AGE NOT DISCLOSED, HETEROSEXUAL, NEW YORK CITY, NY—COMMUNITY ACTIVIST AND AIDS POLICY ANALYST

Even though Glenda had a tumultuous relationship with her family members, Glenda maintains close ties with her siblings. Her mother practiced social work while her father studied in school. Glenda's educational background is in public policy and she earned a master's degree. She was raised on the West Coast but later moved to DC as an adult before moving to New York City. During her time in DC, she learned about HIV criminalization's deleterious effects before being diagnosed with HIV herself.

Glenda considers herself an activist and policy analyst who engages in community-based activism. She writes articles and letters to government officials, attends meetings, and trains other activists in order to help Black communities access AIDS resources. She also advocates for women's representation in AIDS surveillance data and participates in clinical trials for HIV medication.

Glenda's main goal is to end discrimination against HIV-positive individuals, and has experienced multiple forms of discrimination along the way, such as the discrimination she experienced from her landlord. Glenda explains that living as an activist is difficult because she cannot always do things to benefit her own health, such as make doctor's appointments and take HIV medications because she doesn't have the time since she is so engrossed in her activism work.

ISABELLA, 47, HETEROSEXUAL, NEW YORK CITY, NY— COMMUNITY ACTIVIST

Isabella had a troubled upbringing. Her immediate family members abused illicit substances. Her grandmother later intervened and raised her. She then started her trajectory in community-based activism, specifically AIDS activism and prevention, when she was diagnosed with HIV. Isabella eventually completed her bachelor's degree and worked at a major medical research organization. She then participated in HIV surveillance and focused on women's representation in HIV data collection. At the time of the interview, she was in a long-term relationship.

Isabella is a peer advocate who primarily works with Black communities. She empowers women, works with them to improve their self-esteem, help the women prevent themselves from becoming infected with HIV, and facilitates their treatment if infected. In her professional career, she works with incarcerated and post-incarcerated populations. Her occupation provides underprivileged, HIV-positive, or AIDS patients with emotional support and medical and social work access. For example, Isabella helps homeless women transition into positions of economic and financial stability.

Living with HIV, her main motivation is to prevent other women from becoming HIV-positive. However, Isabella suggests that the government poses the biggest challenge for her. In her experience, she does not believe that the government prioritizes Black communities in their research. Furthermore, Isabella believes that AIDS nonprofits should focus on the comorbidities of HIV, such as substance abuse, mental health concerns, diabetes, and cardiovascular disease. In addition, Isabella believes addressing women's self-esteem problems, proper decision making, family planning, and condom use should factor into AIDS interventions.

JASMINE, 51, QUEER, NEW YORK CITY, NY— REINTEGRATION SPECIALIST AND AIDS EDUCATOR

Jasmine was born in New York City. She and her sister were primarily raised by her mother, who worked as an administrative assistant. Her father was in the military. After graduating from high school, Jasmine was the first in her family to graduate from college after majoring in human services. Jasmine is married with children.

Jasmine serves as a reintegration specialist where she educates faith-based communities about HIV-positive women who are reintegrating into society. She also works with health providers, prevention specialists, and parole officers. In addition to her volunteer work, she works full-time.

Jasmine's main goal is to eradicate AIDS stigma, discrimination, and silence and she suggests a number of strategies to do so, such as contributing to lobbying efforts and working with steering committees. Additionally, she organizes meetings and telephone calls, and participates in ad hoc meetings.

Her most effective strategy is sharing stories. She feels that while these strategies might take time, the end results are usually worth it. Jasmine also mentions that it is important to affirm hard work and to remind others about their successes. While Jasmine works tirelessly to eradicate stigma, her main challenge to ending AIDS stigma is access to funding.

JESSICA, 48, HETEROSEXUAL, DETROIT, MI— AIDS CASE MANAGER

Growing up in an upper-middle-class neighborhood, Jessica was raised by her grandmother, who volunteered in homeless shelters and other community organizations throughout her childhood. As a youth, Jessica watched famous speakers on television and realized she wanted to be a public speaker too, but after dropping out of high school, she was incarcerated and rehabilitated for substance abuse. Jessica feels that recovery from substance abuse defines her life. She is divorced with children.

As part of her activism, Jessica chairs a local AIDS advisory board by reviewing protocols for various medications and produces community events. In her activism, she serves multiple underserved populations, including women and LGBTQ+ communities. As a case manager for HIV-positive communities, she works in mobile treatment centers for substance abuse by primarily participating in syringe exchanges.

Jessica's main goal is to give those with HIV hope and to relay the message that HIV is not a death sentence. To do this, Jessica takes a "hands-on" approach to her activism by simply meeting people where they're at and making them feel comfortable. She also dresses causally when she speaks for major events. Jessica encourages individuals to get tested for HIV by announcing testing locations over a loud speaker and asks individuals directly about their sexual behaviors.

JENNIFER, 54, HETEROSEXUAL, WASHINGTON, DC—COMMUNITY ACTIVIST AND AIDS MOTIVATIONAL SPEAKER

Raised in Baton Rouge, Louisiana, Jennifer recalled the impact that Black women had on her upbringing. Not only was she raised in a matriarchal home, she was paired with Black women in a Big Sister, Little Sister program at the YMCA. In this program, Jennifer was exposed to the arts (e.g., museums and dance), and this played a major role in her life. Jennifer is Baptist and was raised in a religious home with strong community ties. However, she faced a series of problems in her youth—she dated a substance abuser and later served prison time—which ultimately culminated in her testing positive for HIV. She then decided to work in AIDS education and advocacy. She first went to work for a needle-exchange program before becoming involved in other forms of advocacy such as AIDS education, safer sex, and healthcare access. In addition to being HIV-positive, she faces a number of other health challenges, but she perseveres in her advocacy. Jennifer has a bachelor's degree, has children, and is in a long-term relationship.

The main goal of Jennifer's work is that she wants to save lives. Jennifer believes that substance abuse and unprotected sexual intercourse are the key drivers of HIV transmission in Black communities. As a needle-exchange advocate, Jennifer works primarily with Black communities, providing services, such as managing a safe-needle exchange; identifying barriers for structurally marginalized groups (e.g., housing, substance abuse, or healthcare); and traveling to individuals' homes to address these specific barriers in their substance abuse treatment. In her needle-exchange work, she describes registering a patient with a particular number of needles if the person provided personal information for the service. In exchange, they would receive a kit that that contains clean needles, cotton balls, Band-Aids, and condoms. Jennifer would also direct clients to HIV testing sites. She gets paid for this work part-time.

JOCELYN, 51, SEXUALITY NOT DISCLOSED, NEW YORK CITY, NY—AIDS EDUCATOR

Jocelyn's family and loved ones motivate her activism work and her grandmother and daughter inspire her. Her parents worked as journalists and documented the civil rights era. Jocelyn's bisexual partner passed away because of AIDS-related complications during the onset of the AIDS epidemic. She described this death as "heart-wrenching" because he was one "of the best lovers of life." Though she lost her partner, she had children. These factors impacted how Jocelyn developed her activist identity and drove her to join AIDS organizations.

Jocelyn's activism focuses on community education and cultural performances for Black women and Black men who have sex with men. Jocelyn works with various committees which produce conferences, panel discussions, interfaith discussions, and rallies that specifically address AIDS. In this work, Jocelyn raises awareness around AIDS and same-sex sexualities through performance art. For example, she "blesses" condoms, female condoms, and safer sex kits. She also writes religious "passages" that bless sexuality.

The core of her activism is a need to address the struggles of Black women. However, Jocelyn faces multiple challenges in this work. Jocelyn encounters negative attitudes from those within her local communities because some people negatively judge her for the work that she does. For example, she believes that she has a reputation for being divisive. She reports that she earned this perception from her local Black churches. Not only does she believe that Black churches prevent effective AIDS education in communities, she also believes that its leaders prevent women and gay men from assuming leadership positions. Ultimately, she wishes for the Black Church to, as she put it, "completely change."

JULIET, 52, HETEROSEXUAL, BATON ROUGE, LA— COMMUNITY ACTIVIST AND AIDS MOTIVATIONAL SPEAKER

Juliet grew up witnessing a significant amount of domestic violence between her parents. She believes that once her parents separated, she emulated her mother's frequent dating patterns and experiences of domestic violence along with alcohol and drug dependency. After discovering she was HIV-positive, Juliet became inspired by the work of other AIDS activists and decided to engage in AIDS advocacy work herself. She also has two sons and a deceased daughter.

Juliet described her life as an activist as, "a life I have to live. Like I say, it gives me the opportunity to stay in the forefront, try to learn new things, try to keep up with what's going on. I do what I can to help other people." Juliet's activism focuses on community outreach and public speaking. She primarily works with Black and Latinx gay, bisexual, and trans-identified men. Juliet passes out flyers providing AIDS information, helps organize and attends fundraisers, tests individuals for HIV, and hires other motivational speakers. She works with schools, churches, and other institutions to provide safer sex and AIDS education.

When discussing how she became involved in AIDS education, Juliet explained, "I get out here because I don't want no one else to walk in my shoes." After her HIV diagnosis, Juliet found that sharing her story was instrumental to raising AIDS awareness in others. For example, after one of her talks where she discussed how she contracted HIV and her experiences with the virus, several young women from the audience approached Juliet and expressed how emotional they became during her presentation as they realized they would not have thought she was HIV-positive and that they cannot judge an individual's HIV status based on appearances. This motivated the women to practice safer sex and Juliet continues to remain in contact with these women.

JUNE, 53, HETEROSEXUAL, NEW YORK CITY, NY— AIDS EDUCATOR AND AIDS MOTIVATIONAL SPEAKER

June had a religious upbringing and was raised Methodist by her mother in Cincinnati. While she was raised in a religious home, it was her pastor who encouraged her to look beyond the religion to focus on her spirituality. She used the Bible as her spiritual guide and focused on the teachings of Jesus Christ. An entertainer, she is single with two adult children. June became involved in AIDS activism work when she was diagnosed with HIV.

June is an AIDS motivational speaker, runs an AIDS ministry, and works to convene AIDS service and health service organizations. She mostly works within Black communities. June is passionate about addressing misconceptions about HIV transmission and providing safer sex education and paraphernalia. June explained that her main message is "Love. . . . Letting people know that your life is worthwhile." June primarily volunteers her services and generally volunteers her efforts without compensation as she works full time in the music industry.

In the end, June just wants to get "people to change how they feel about themselves and make better choices." She provides people with information about HIV transmission and believes that combatting myths about HIV within Black communities is the first step toward reducing rates in these communities. June also works to address AIDS stigma and the shame those with HIV may feel about their diagnosis. June maintains that this shame prevents individuals from learning about HIV and their own risk-taking behaviors. Finally, as a college graduate, June values education. She does not believe that the government invests enough money into educating others about the virus and providing safer sex resources, which would have a major impact on reducing infection rates in Black communities.

LANETTA, 60, HETEROSEXUAL, MILWAUKEE, WI— AIDS SUPPORT GROUP FACILITATOR, AIDS EDUCATOR, AND LOBBYIST

Lanetta grew up in foster care. After her placement in several homes, a family adopted her. While her family was politically active, they typically limited their conversations around sexuality. As a parent, Lanetta works to rectify this because she believes that her children should have accurate information about sexuality. In her spare time, she spends time with her children and grandchildren.

Lanetta works full time and part of her work consists of educating Black youth about sex. In her activism, Lanetta designs curriculum for high school students, and she educates her students on chronic disease experiences and other STIs. Lanetta wants to, as she explained, "continue to train young adults and youth, give them an introduction to behavioral science and what it is and where it might fit in their future career plan." She stresses that this information needs to be sound and unbiased.

As someone who values education and has some collegiate experience, Lanetta wants to dispel myths about HIV. When Lanetta was young, she worked with HIV-positive artists who later died of AIDS. While she did not have concerns about hugging these artists, other people around them did not know that physical contact alone did not spread HIV. Lanetta also wants to dispel the myth that there is a cure to HIV. She believes that that education helps others stay informed and this information can help make communities more inclusive.

LATRICE, 48, HETEROSEXUAL, DETROIT, MI— COMMUNITY ACTIVIST AND AIDS EDUCATOR

Latrice grew up going to church every Sunday with her mother. Although she still believes in God and Jesus, she does not identify as a deeply religious person. Latrice is single with three adult daughters. She has some college experience, but did not graduate, and is unemployed and engages in unpaid AIDS advocacy work.

Latrice became engaged in AIDS advocacy because she firmly believed that if one is infected with HIV, they need to understand the virus and its impact on the body. Latrice's activism focuses primarily on education and peer mentorship for HIV-positive women as she has experienced the positive effects of being in a support group with other HIV-positive women herself. She works with HIV-positive mothers, their children, and gay and bisexual men. She fundraises for social services, conducts HIV testing, and distributes safer sex paraphernalia. Maintaining that she pours her heart into her community, Latrice relishes the opportunity to give back to those in need.

The primary challenges Latrice faces in her work all pertain to funding. Beyond the fact that competition for more funds reduces collaboration and programmatic innovation, additional funding could serve a number of purposes, such as providing gift card incentives to encourage testing. However, in the end, she believes that the biggest challenge is accurate AIDS education. Latrice believes that communities need to understand how the virus is transmitted and impacts the body and how to obtain support/outreach. According to Latrice, this education is not done in the classroom, but, rather, HIV-positive individuals must seek out information on their own and advocate for their health.

MARVA, 30, HETEROSEXUAL, NEW YORK CITY, NY— DIRECTOR OF A HEALTH ORGANIZATION

Coming from a Southern background, Marva was raised in a working-class family in New York City. Although her parents did not complete college, she earned two master's degrees. She also is in a long-term relationship, and she does not have children. Marva is deeply spiritual and distinguishes her belief system from church worship and religious ritual. Identifying as spiritual, a belief in a "God-given" purpose and divine incidences, or "miracles," drives her work. Ultimately, these spiritualist beliefs influence her activism, especially her interaction with younger communities.

Given her relationship with spirituality and youth groups, Marva participates in community activism in schools and in Black churches. In addition to engaging in youth outreach, Marva worked as an outreach program facilitator and provided cultural-sensitivity training for clergy members. As an extension of her church work, her program also engages in homeless shelter outreach, provides AIDS education, and connects individuals to services. In addition, Marva helps unhoused populations access the support and resources offered by Black churches.

Based on Marva's experiences with activism, Marva wants to alleviate stigma and provide support and resources. To do so, she suggests an end to mass incarceration because it contributes to how AIDS negatively impacts Black communities, especially Black women. As someone who is diagnosed with HIV, the primary goal of her work is to serve as a role model to others with HIV and help empower them to find the strength to be "able to stand up and [say] look, 'I have this disease, it's not taking over my life; it's actually a part of me.'"

PEGGY, 57, QUEER, DENVER, CO— AIDS EDUCATOR AND CONSULTANT

Peggy's family has been based in Colorado for several generations. Growing up in a religious home, she identifies as spiritual, is not married, but is in a relationship, and has co-parented four children. She has an associate's degree. When her friends began to die from AIDS-related complications, Peggy went to work in AIDS advocacy. She first provided AIDS education in juvenile detention centers and then expanded her program to include gay and bisexual men of color.

Peggy's activism focuses on education, and she is employed as a curriculum development consultant for a charter school and its school board. In this curriculum, she focuses on HIV prevention that targets teenagers of color, namely through safer sex education and learning sexual negotiation. Additionally, Peggy focuses on building trust with the adolescents that she teaches and develops a culturally informed curriculum.

The death of several friends not only served as the impetus of Peggy's AIDS activism but it also helps motivate her to continue her work even in the face of adversity. Peggy describes how a lack of funding increases competition and decreases a lack of cooperation and comradery among local community AIDS activists. She believes that not enough funding goes to HIV prevention, and, although this is her biggest challenge, she feels that compassion and patience are the two primary qualities AIDS activists must have, and these qualities ground and focus her AIDS advocacy work.

ROSE, 42, QUEER, BROOKLYN, NY—MEDIA ACTIVIST

Rose's family originated from the West Indies and settled in New York City. Her mother owned a small business and her father worked for a manufacturing company. While her family was not involved in activism, her mother emphasized civic participation and involved herself in community politics, especially West-Indian politics. Her family is largely Christian, but Rose identifies as spiritual. After attending high school, Rose went on to earn both a bachelor's and a master's degree.

Rose works as a filmmaker and considers herself a media activist and produces films to promote visibility, social justice, and inclusion. The goal of her activism work is to encourage dialogue and education, and to reform the status quo.

Rose was motivated to engage in activism because of the death of a loved one. In her activism work, she encounters multiple challenges, mainly a lack of funding and resistance to AIDS education. Among other concerns, Rose believes that granting organizations neither believe in the importance of addressing AIDS in Black communities, nor do they acknowledge the work that Black communities have already done to address AIDS. Additionally, Rose encounters resistance to AIDS education from educated Black women as they usually do not believe they can become infected with HIV. Likewise, she believes that other Black individuals need to practice safer sex and hold themselves accountable for their sexual practices. To address these issues, Rose explains that we need to incorporate HIV testing and safer sex into our everyday dialogue with doctors, pastors, and other individuals.

ROXSAN, 65, HETEROSEXUAL, DALLAS, TX—EVANGELIST, AIDS EDUCATOR, AIDS MOTIVATIONAL SPEAKER

Roxsan is divorced with one daughter and two grandchildren, whom she raised. Roxsan grew up in a small town in Louisiana and was raised in an Evangelical home. Her parents worked as architects and strictly monitored her activities. As a teenager, she developed several skills, including auto maintenance and cosmetology. Roxsan eventually went to college but left without finishing, and eventually became a high-ranking executive at a national bank. She then contracted HIV, which changed her career and life trajectory.

Roxsan now works as a peer educator and primarily works directly with school boards, politicians, individuals, and lobbyists. Key aspects of her advocacy efforts are to secure housing for those with HIV and solicit funding for HIV medication. Roxsan mostly engages in fundraising and has even met with members of Congress to advocate for expanding HIV services and resources. Roxsan's activism targets low-income Black and Latinx communities and she also wants to connect those in need with resources and support.

Roxsan faces her own health issues that challenge her activism work. Roxsan has a history of chronic pain and other chronic health issues in addition to HIV. She has difficulty accessing her medications. Roxsan believes she lost Ryan White program benefits when she moved to a Southern state, and, as a result, she struggles with Medicare, co-pays, and other expenses. She also has to be aware of her own ailments, and she has to know how to navigate health care systems. Understanding the difficulty that people have in accessing health care, Roxsan is motivated to work to create change and enhance access to medicine and health support resources.

RUBY, 49, HETEROSEXUAL, SAN DIEGO, CA—COMMUNITY ACTIVIST AND AIDS MOTIVATIONAL SPEAKER

Ruby grew up primarily in Northern California with her parents, but she also lived in Hawaii and New Jersey for brief periods of time. Her mother was from Panama and a Black Panther. Her father worked as a seaman. When she was a child, she faced ostracism because of her skin color and her clothing.

Eventually, her mother moved her and her seven brothers, who she described as "very overprotective," into a house where they were largely self-sufficient. She would eventually earn her bachelor's degree. Ruby is single and has children.

Ruby volunteers as a community activist and motivational speaker. She also organizes emotional support groups for Black women in her church community and runs an AIDS ministry. These support groups help these women understand how HIV impacts their lives, their families, and their access to social services.

She believes that people from small towns—especially individuals with HIV—should voice their experiences and concerns with the government so they understand the lack of resources and support that people in small towns receive. She also notes that funding is very competitive and that a number of structurally marginalized groups consistently compete for the few funding opportunities available.

RUE, 45, QUEER, BOSTON, MA—COMMUNITY ACTIVIST

Growing up middle-class, Rue's mother worked in social services. All of her family members were nurses, doctors, and teachers who instilled, as she described, a "voluntarist ethos" within Rue, especially as it centers church and community service. Additionally, Rue notes that this ethos was part of a cultural obligation to support her community members.

Rue considers herself a community advocate that coordinates efforts to highlight Black disability issues within AIDS discourse and outreach. Working in the context of predominately White-led queer organizations and health-focused organizations, her activism largely targets Black communities. Similarly, she also engages in media activism where she develops visibility campaigns for university audiences and applies her master's degree in media studies to create AIDS educational material. Rue worked as a program manager and applies her education to a nonprofit that provides legal services for structurally marginalized groups.

Rue believes that her identity as a Black lesbian motivates her activism, however, her racial identity takes precedence over other identities and experiences. She mentions that her family raised her to understand the importance of community advocacy, especially because her mother and her extended family focused on community service.

Rue believes that the Black Church's inability to promote sexually inclusive education, and gender-inclusive education, stymie her activism efforts. To address these issues, Rue maintains that the Black Church should stress sexual inclusivity, especially in respect to its LGBTQ+ communities. Finally, she suggests that men's groups in Black churches should identify and discuss issues relating to sexual violence and crime.

SANDY, 48, HETEROSEXUAL, NEW YORK CITY, NY— COMMUNITY ACTIVIST

Sandy grew up in New York City, and she was raised in a family that valued activism and a college education. Her mother worked as a mammographer and focused primarily on women's health, including breast cancer and sexual health. Her father was involved in community initiatives. In addition to her parents' activism, Sandy developed empathy for what she described as "slightly different" individuals through her interaction with her physically disabled grandfather. Sandy also earned her master's degree.

As part of her activism, Sandy is a community advocate for youth who navigate criminal justice or foster care systems and for families who were impacted by AIDS or substance abuse. In addition to her job as a social worker, she also serves on a major national AIDS taskforce, and through this work, she coordinates grants to invest in an AIDS education program that educates Black leadership.

At the core of her activism is Sandy's desire to see a world where she does not have to test teenagers for HIV. However, she faces a number of challenges to achieving this goal. For example, Sandy believes that although AIDS is discussed more frequently in Black communities because of Magic Johnson, gay and bisexual men are still stigmatized, and individuals blame down low culture for the increase in the rates of HIV among Black women. She also believes that Black communities need more mentoring programs for younger groups. Furthermore, another challenge is education, because, for example, some older women believe that they do not need to practice safer sex because they are no longer able to reproduce.

To address these challenges, Sandy stresses the importance of educating higher-risk groups, especially when they live in tight-knit communities.

SHANICE, 59, HETEROSEXUAL, NEW YORK CITY, NY— COMMUNITY ACTIVIST AND AIDS MOTIVATIONAL SPEAKER

Shanice came from a close family. Her father was an alderman and her mother, a housewife. Additionally, Shanice was the eldest of seven siblings and was largely responsible for nurturing her siblings and cousins. Although her family was not religious, Shanice found herself attracted to religion and spirituality and grew to become deeply religious. Shanice has some college education, but she did not complete her degree. Shanice is single with three adult children, including one who works as a college professor and one who works as a police officer.

Motivated to provide AIDS education and support by her own HIV diagnosis, Shanice works as a peer educator and runs her church's AIDS ministry. In her ministry, she works diligently to ensure that she provides congregants and community members with accurate AIDS education, HIV prevention information, and support. Shanice also works with those who have experienced substance abuse, mental health concerns, and those who live below the poverty level. She works part-time at a health services organization.

Shanice believes that education is the key to reducing HIV rates in Black communities. She is constantly in training as she believes that medical technology is rapidly advancing, so she wants to ensure she keeps up with the most up-to-date AIDS information and resources. Although she is deeply engaged in the Black Church, Shanice finds that the abstinence-only education advocated by Black churches, including her own, prevents people from understanding their own risk or how to protect themselves when they do engage in sexual activity.

SHAY, 56, HETEROSEXUAL, SOUTH CAROLINA—
COUNSELOR, COMMUNITY ACTIVIST,
AND AIDS EDUCATOR

Shay has been engaged in AIDS activism work since the early 1990s and sees this work as an important part of her identity. Deeply religious, Shay is single with one adult child.

Much of Shay's AIDS activism work is unpaid as she helps women of color advocate for themselves, raise their self-esteem, develop personal responsibility, and hold themselves accountable. Shay is engaged in numerous types of activism work. She works in transitional housing, and, as part of her job, provides additional support around HIV testing and treatment for substance abuse disorders. As part of her volunteer work, Shay works at an AIDS ministry at her church and also facilitates support groups for those newly diagnosed with HIV to cope with the illness and to find support. She also lobbies members of Congress by writing letters and reaching out online.

Shay values education and has a bachelor's degree. Shay believes that knowledge empowers individuals and leads to positive outcomes. She maintains that many in the public have negative misconceptions about those with HIV and that these stigmas contribute to the high rates of HIV in Black communities. In addition to providing accurate and up-to-date AIDS education and prevention information, Shay argues that one of the primary ways to help reduce rates of HIV in Black communities is to provide additional funding for further community outreach and to support safer sex campaigns.

TAMMY, 37, HETEROSEXUAL, PHILADELPHIA, PA— AIDS RESEARCHER AND AIDS EDUCATOR

Tammy was born in Florida, and spent a good part of her youth moving around with her family to different communities in the South before moving to New Orleans for college, where she graduated with her bachelor's degree. While her parents were not politically engaged, her grandparents were politically active. For example, her grandmother worked on a mayoral campaign and photographed local politicians. Tammy was raised in a deeply religious home and is not only the child of a preacher, but is also a granddaughter of a preacher and "the niece of about 15 preachers." After learning about Ryan White—a young boy who was not allowed to attend school because he had AIDS—she became interested in social justice and community activism. Tammy now sees activism and social justice as important parts of her identity and her life. She is married and does not have children.

As part of her activism, Tammy worked as a researcher and AIDS educator in an AIDS service organization that primarily works with communities of color and gay, bisexual, and trans men who have sex with men. Initially, Tammy tested individuals for HIV antibodies, but, later, Tammy refocused her work toward completing administrative tasks and even engaging in research—focusing on testing requirements and procedures. Tammy is involved in local community politics. She also wants to increase Black men's representation in community groups and in AIDS research and AIDS-related politics.

The primary motivation behind Tammy's activism work is her desire to live in a fair and just world; however, there are multiple challenges that she faces as part of her activism. For example, she finds it difficult to connect with other activists and finds that sometimes there are barriers between herself and other activists. She feels these barriers limit her ability to reach areas of the community and broaden her advocacy work. HIV-negative, Tammy believes that we can improve AIDS advocacy work by creating better unity between HIV-positive and HIV-negative activists.

TARA, 59, HETEROSEXUAL, OAKLAND, CA—
COMMUNITY ACTIVIST

Coming from a family that focused on public health and nursing, Tara's family emphasized a culture of care. Her family was educated and Tara was no exception as she went on to college and received her bachelor's degree. Tara sees AIDS activism as part of her broader concern for women's health equity and social justice. She also sees AIDS as a human rights issue. She is single and has three children.

Tara considers herself a community advocate and she organizes events for Black women, such as HIV testing events and HIV education days. As an executive director of a reproductive rights nonprofit, she works full time to address these issues while also fundraising for HIV nonprofits.

Tara notes that inequities are "where disease lives" and finds that HIV-positive women face greater cultural stigma because, for many, HIV is associated with sex and sexuality. Tara acknowledges, "the courage it takes for women to say publicly that they are HIV-positive. That just, every single time, it floors me, because I know how people judge and the stigma associated." She is motivated by a need to help encourage women to have more autonomy over their bodies. Tara notes women face structural inequity on multiple fronts, including their reproductive rights, and is concerned with the rights of women nationally and globally.

TRACY, 36, HETEROSEXUAL, PHILADELPHIA, PA—
COMMUNITY ACTIVIST AND AIDS EDUCATOR

Tracy grew up in a family that avoided any discussion of sex or sexuality. Her parents were deeply religious—her mother was Catholic and her father, Baptist. As a result of her conservative religious upbringing, she had a limited understanding of sex and sexuality and sought information on her own. Eventually she went on to college and received her bachelor's degree. Her experiences with her family and their conservative nature drew her to work in sexual health education. Initially, her family was not supportive of her work, but her family eventually acquiesced and became more comfortable with conversations around sexuality. When she realized individuals felt comfortable discussing sexuality with her, she worked to provide clear HIV messaging, something she felt was lacking in Black communities.

Tracy works full time as an event planner and engages in volunteer AIDS advocacy work, including HIV testing, outreach, peer mentorship, and HIV prevention. Her activism primarily focuses on women of color who lack financial resources, have criminal backgrounds, or reside in transitional housing. Tracy believes that, "You would definitely need empathy to understand their pain" and believes that this empathy is an important part of her activism.

The primary goal of Tracy's activism work is to ensure that communities have an accurate understanding of AIDS. She believes that the media greatly influences how communities understand AIDS. Although the media is an important institution that relays information to large audiences, Tracy believes that many media outlets often convey inaccurate information, so individuals should be sure to educate themselves about HIV, particularly as new science and research emerges.

VIRGINIA, 50, HETEROSEXUAL, PHILADELPHIA, PA— AIDS EDUCATOR

Virginia has strong family ties and was raised by her grandmother. She described the emotional support she received from family members when she dealt with the death of her son. She became involved in AIDS activism when she was diagnosed with HIV and had a close family member who passed away from an AIDS-related illness. Virginia attributes this death to the lack of community resources and support and she wants to ensure that others receive adequate support. She joined an AIDS service organization that provides access to AIDS education and resources.

Virginia has an associate's degree and works in a national nonprofit as an AIDS educator. Understanding the many social issues that influence experiences with AIDS, Virginia provides education, training, and resources to address issues such as housing disparities, educational inequities, mass incarceration, substance abuse, and the digital divide in Black and other structurally marginalized communities. Her main goal is to see a generation free from AIDS.

Virginia argues that individuals stigmatize HIV-positive individuals, and this contributes to multiple misunderstandings, especially because some members of Black communities still believe that AIDS is a "gay White disease." To combat this issue, Virginia maintains that it is important to share stories and address misinformation.

References

ACT UP NY/ Women AIDS Book Group. 1999. *Women, AIDS, and Activism.* Boston: South End Press.

Anderson, Cheryl. 2016. "The Song of Songs: Redeeming Gender Constructions in the Age of AIDS." In *Womanist Interpretations of the Bible,* edited by Gay L. Byron and Vanessa Lovelace, 73–92. Atlanta: SBL Press.

Andrasfay, Theresa, and Noreen Goldman. 2021. "Reductions in 2020 US Life Expectancy Due to COVID-19 and the Disproportionate Impact on the Black and Latino Populations." *Proceedings of the National Academy of Sciences* 118, no. 5: e2014746118.

Armon-Jones, Claire. 1986. "The Thesis of Constructionism." In *The Social Construction of Emotions,* edited by Rom Harre, 32–56. Oxford: Blackwell.

Assari, Shervin. 2017. "Combined Racial and Gender Differences in the Long-Term Predictive Role of Education on Depressive Symptoms and Chronic Medical Conditions." *Journal of Racial and Ethnic Health Disparities* 4, no. 3: 385–396.

Assari, Shervin, Ehsan Moazen Zadah, Cleopatra H. Caldwell, and Marc A. Zimmerman 2017. "Racial Discrimination during Adolescence Predicts Mental Health Deterioration in Adulthood: Gender Differences among Blacks." *Frontiers in Public Health,* 5: 104.

Bacchus, Denise N. A., and Lynn C. Holley. 2005. "Spirituality as a Coping Resource: The Experiences of Professional Black Women." *Journal of Ethnic and Cultural Diversity in Social Work* 13, no. 4: 65–84.

Baker-Fletcher, Karen. 2017. *Sisters of Dust, Sisters of Spirit: Womanist Wordings on God and Creation.* Minneapolis: Fortress Press.

Baltrus, Peter T., Megan Douglas, Chaohua Li, Lee S. Caplan, Mitchell Blount, Dominic Mack, and Anne H. Gaglioti. 2021. "Percentage of Black Population and Primary Care Shortage Areas Associated with Higher COVID-19 Case and Death Rates in Georgia Counties." *Southern Medical Journal* 114, no. 2: 57.

Banks–Wallace, JoAnne. 1998. "Emancipatory Potential of Storytelling in a Group." *Image: The Journal of Nursing Scholarship* 30, no. 1: 17–22.

Banks-Wallace, JoAnne. 2000. "Womanist Ways of Knowing: Theoretical Considerations for Research with African American Women." *Advances in Nursing Science* 22, no. 3: 33–45.

Beauboeuf-Lafontant, Tamara. 2002. "A Womanist Experience of Caring: Understanding the Pedagogy of Exemplary Black Women Teachers." *The Urban Review* 34, no. 1: 71–86.

Beauboeuf-Lafontant, Tamara. 2005. "Womanist Lessons for Reinventing Teaching." *Journal of Teacher Education* 56, no. 5: 436–445.

Berger, Michele Tracy. 2010. *Workable Sisterhood: The Political Journey of Stigmatized Women with HIV/AIDS*. Princeton: Princeton University Press.

Bibbins-Domingo, Kirsten. 2020. "This Time Must Be Different: Disparities during the COVID-19 Pandemic." *Annals of Internal Medicine* 173, no. 3: 233–234.

Bogart, Laura M., and Sheryl Thorburn. 2005. "Are HIV/AIDS Conspiracy Beliefs a Barrier to HIV Prevention among African Americans?" *Journal of Acquired Immune Deficiency Syndromes* 38, no. 2: 213–218.

Bond, Lisa, Darrell P. Wheeler, Gregorio A. Millett, Archana Bodas LaPollo, Lee F. Carson, and Adrian Liau. 2009. "Black Men Who Have Sex with Men and the Association of Down-Low Identity with HIV Risk Behavior." *American Journal of Public Health* 99, no. S1: S92–S95.

Bowleg, Lisa. 2008. "When Black+ Lesbian+ Woman ≠ Black Lesbian Woman: The Methodological Challenges of Qualitative and Quantitative Intersectionality Research." *Sex Roles* 59, no. 5: 312–325.

Bowleg, Lisa, Torsten B. Neilands, Loni Philip Tabb, Gary J. Burkholder, David J. Malebranche, and Jeanne M. Tschann. 2014. "Neighborhood Context and Black Heterosexual Men's Sexual HIV Risk Behaviors." *AIDS and Behavior* 18, no. 11: 2207–2218.

Braxton, Nikia D., Delia L. Lang, Jessica M. Sales, Gina M. Wingood, and Ralph J. DiClemente. 2007. "The Role of Spirituality in Sustaining the Psychological Well-Being of HIV-Positive Black Women." *Women & Health* 46, no. 2–3: 113–129.

Brijnath, Bianca. 2007. "It's About Time: Engendering AIDS in Africa." *Culture, Health, and Sexuality* 9, no. 4: 371–386.

Broaddus, Michelle R., Wayne J. DiFranceisco, Jeffrey A. Kelly, Janet S. St. Lawrence, Yuri A. Amirkhanian, and Julia D. Dickson-Gomez. 2015. "Social Media Use and High-Risk Sexual Behavior among Black Men Who Have Sex with Men: A Three-City Study." *AIDS and Behavior* 19, no. 2: 90–97.

Brooks, Ronald A., Vincent C. Allen Jr., Rotrease Regan, Matt G. Mutchler, Ramon Cervantes-Tadeo, and Sung-Jae Lee. 2018. "HIV/AIDS Conspiracy Beliefs and Intention to Adopt Preexposure Prophylaxis among Black Men Who Have Sex with Men in Los Angeles." *International Journal of STDS & AIDS* 29, no. 4: 375–381.

Brown, R. Khari, and Ronald E. Brown. 2003. "Faith and Works: Church-Based Social Capital Resources and African American Political Activism." *Social Forces* 82, no. 2: 617–641.

Buhuro, Danielle J. 2018. "Transforming Trauma into Trust: A Prophetic Model of CPE Supervision in the Age of #Black Lives Matter." *Reflective Practice: Formation and Supervision in Ministry* 38: 154–164.

Calabrese, Sarah K., Valerie A. Earnshaw, Kristen Underhill, Nathan B. Hansen, and John F. Dovidio. 2014. "The Impact of Patient Race on Clinical Decisions Related to Prescribing HIV Pre-Exposure Prophylaxis (PrEP): Assumptions about Sexual Risk Compensation and Implications for Access." *AIDS and Behavior* 18, no. 2: 226–240.

Campbell, Jacquelyn C., and Karen L. Soeken. 1999. "Forced Sex and Intimate Partner Violence: Effects on Women's Risk and Women's Health." *Violence Against Women* 5, no. 9: 1017–1035.

Carlton-LaNey, Iris. 2001. *African American Leadership: An Empowerment Tradition in Social Welfare History.* District of Columbia: NASW Press.

Carlton-LaNey, Iris. 1999. "African American Social Work Pioneers' Response to Need." *Social Work* 44, no. 4: 311–321.

Carrillo Rowe, Aimee, and Francesca T. Royster. 2017. "Loving Transgressions: Queer of Color Bodies, Affective Ties, Transformative Community." *Journal of Lesbian Studies* 21, no. 3: 243–253.

Center for Disease Control. 2021a. "HIV among Transgender People." Last modified April 15, 2021. https://www.cdc.gov/hiv/group/gender/transgender/index.html.

Center for Disease Control. 2021b. "HIV among African Americans." Last modified January 20, 2021. https://www.cdc.gov/hiv/group/racialethnic/africanamericans /index.html.

Chambers, Lori Ann. 2018. "Because She Cares: Re-Membering, Re-Finding, and Poetically Retelling Narratives of HIV Caring Work with, for and by African Women Living with HIV." PhD diss., Macmaster University.

Chandler, Rasheeta, Dominique Guillaume, Andrea G. Parker, Amber Mack, Jill Hamilton, Jemea Dorsey, and Natalie D. Hernandez. 2021. "The Impact of COVID-19 among Black Women: Evaluating Perspectives and Sources of Information." *Ethnicity & Health* 26, no. 1: 80–93.

Charmaz, Kathy. 2002. *Constructing Grounded Theory.* Thousand Oaks: Sage Publications.

Cho, Sumi, Kimberlé Williams Crenshaw, and Leslie McCall. 2013. "Toward a Field of Intersectionality Studies: Theory, Applications, and Praxis." *Signs: Journal of Women in Culture and Society* 38, no. 4: 785–810.

Choo, Hae Yeon, and Myra Marx Ferree. 2010. "Practicing Intersectionality in Sociological Research: A Critical Analysis of Inclusions, Interactions, and Institutions in the Study of Inequalities." *Sociological Theory* 28, no. 2: 129–149.

Chun, Jennifer Jihye, George Lipsitz, and Young Shin. 2013. "Intersectionality as a Social Movement Strategy: Asian Immigrant Women Advocates." *Signs: Journal of Women in Culture and Society* 38, no. 4: 917–940.

Cloy, Cherita Yvonne. 2016. "Exploring Meaningful Experiences of Black Women with HIV: A Qualitative Study of Relational Care Practices and Spirituality." PhD diss., Boston University.

Cohen, Cathy J. 1999. *The Boundaries of Blackness: AIDS and the Breakdown of Black Politics.* Chicago: University of Chicago Press.

Collins, Patricia Hill. 1996. "What's in a Name? Womanism, Black Feminism, and Beyond." *Journal of Black Studies and Research* 26, no. 1: 9–17.

Collins, Patricia Hill. 2000. "Gender, Black Feminism, and Black Political Economy." *The Annals of the American Academy of Political and Social Science* 568, no. 1: 41–53.

Collins, Patricia Hill. 2002. *Black Feminist Thought: Knowledge, Consciousness, and the Politics of Empowerment*. London: Routledge.

Cone, James. 1996. *From God of the Oppressed*. Durham: Duke University Press.

Corea, Gena. 1992. *The Invisible Epidemic: The Story of Women and AIDS*. New York: Perennial Press.

Crenshaw, Kimberlé. 2018 [1989]. *Demarginalizing the Intersection of Race and Sex: A Black Feminist Critique of Antidiscrimination Doctrine, Feminist Theory, and Antiracist Politics*. London: Routledge.

Crooks, Natasha, Barbara King, Audrey Tluczek, and Jessica McDermott Sales. 2019. "The Process of Becoming a Sexual Black Woman: A Grounded Theory Study." *Perspectives on Sexual and Reproductive Health* 51, no. 1: 17–25.

Dalmida, Safiya George, Marcia McDonnell Holstad, Colleen DiIorio, and Gary Laderman. 2012. "The Meaning and Use of Spirituality among African American Women Living with HIV/AIDS." *Western Journal of Nursing Research* 34, no. 6: 736–765.

Dalton, Harlon L. 1989. "AIDS in Blackface." *Daedalus* 118, no. 3: 205–227.

Dandridge, Rita B. 2004. *Black Women's Activism: Reading African American Women's Historical Romances*. Bern: Peter Lang.

Davis, Angela. 1981. "Reflections on the Black Woman's Role in the Community of Slaves." *The Black Scholar* 12, no. 6: 2–15.

Dill, Bonnie Thornton. 1979. *Across the Boundaries of Race and Class: An Exploration of the Relationship between Work and Family among Black Female Domestic Servants*. New York: Garland Press.

Douglas, Kelly Brown. 2018 [2003]. *Sexuality and the Black Church: A Womanist Perspective*. Maryknoll, Orbis Books.

Duran, Jane. 2010. "African NGO's and Womanism: Microcredit and Self-Help." *Journal of African American Studies* 14, no. 2: 171–180.

Durr, Marlese, and Adia M. Harvey Wingfield. 2011. "Keep Your 'N' in Check: African American Women and the Interactive Effects of Etiquette and Emotional Labor." *Critical Sociology* 37, no. 5: 557–571.

Dworkin, Shari L., Theresa Exner, Rita Melendez, Susie Hoffman, and Anke A. Ehrhardt. 2006. "Revisiting "Success": Posttrial Analysis of a Gender-Specific HIV/STD Prevention Intervention." *AIDS and Behavior* 10, no. 1: 41–51.

Dyson, Michael Eric. 2008. *The Michael Eric Dyson Reader*. Hachette: UK.

Exner, Theresa M., Shari L. Dworkin, Susie Hoffman, and Anke A. Ehrhardt. 2003. "Beyond the Male Condom: The Evolution of Gender-Specific HIV Interventions for Women." *Annual Review of Sex Research* 14, no. 1: 114–136.

Felmlee, Diane & Sprecher, Susan. 2006. "Love." In *Handbook of the Sociology of Emotions*, edited by Jan E. Stets and Jonathan H. Turner, 389–409. New York: Springer Press.

Fletcher, Faith, Lucy Annang Ingram, Jelani Kerr, Meredith Buchberg, Libby Bogdan-Lovis, and Sean Philpott-Jones. 2016. "She Told Them, 'Oh That Bitch

Got AIDS': Experiences of Multilevel HIV/AIDS-Related Stigma among African American Women Living with HIV/AIDS in the South." *AIDS Patient Care and STDs* 30, no. 7: 349–356.

Floyd-Thomas, Stacey M. 2006. *Mining the Motherlode: Methods in Womanist Ethics.* Cleveland: Pilgrim Press.

Fogel, Catherine Ingram, and Michael Belyea. 1999. "The Lives of Incarcerated Women: Violence, Substance Abuse, and at Risk for HIV." *Journal of the Association of Nurses in AIDS Care* 10, no. 6: 66–74.

Ford, Chandra L., Kathryn D. Whetten, Susan A. Hall, Jay S. Kaufman, and Angela D. Thrasher. 2007. "Black Sexuality, Social Construction, and Research Targeting 'The Down Low' ('The DL')." *Annals of Epidemiology* 17, no. 3: 209–216.

Frederick, Marla. 2003. *Between Sundays: Black Women and Everyday Struggles of Faith.* Berkeley: University of California Press.

French, Bryana H. 2013. "More Than Jezebels and Freaks: Exploring How Black Girls Navigate Sexual Coercion and Sexual Scripts." *Journal of African American Studies* 17, no. 1: 35–50.

Friedan, Betty. 2010 [1963]. *The Feminine Mystique.* New York: W. W. Norton & Company.

Friedman, Samuel R., Hannah L. F. Cooper, and Andrew H. Osborne. 2009. "Structural and Social Contexts of HIV Risk among African Americans." *American Journal of Public Health* 99, no. 6: 1002–1008.

Froyum, Carissa M. 2010. "The Reproduction of Inequalities through Emotional Capital: The Case of Socializing Low-Income Black Girls." *Qualitative Sociology* 33, no. 1: 37–54.

Fullilove, Mindy Thompson, Robert E. Fullilove III, Katherine Haynes, and Shirley Gross. 1990. "Black Women and AIDS Prevention: A View towards Understanding the Gender Rules." *Journal of Sex Research* 27, no. 1: 47–64.

Gaines, Kevin. 2006. *Uplifting the Race: Black Leadership, Politics, and Culture in the Twentieth century.* Chapel Hill: UNC Press Books.

Gamson, William. 1992. *Talking Politics.* Cambridge: Cambridge Publishing.

Garza, Alicia. 2016. *Who Do You Serve, Who Do You Protect? Police Violence and Resistance in the United States.* Chicago: Haymarket Books.

Giddens, Anthony. 1996. "Affluence, Poverty and the Idea of a Post–Scarcity Society." *Development and Change* 27, no. 2: 365–377.

Gilkes, Cheryl T. 1980. Holding Back the Ocean with a Broom: Black Women and Community Work." In *The Black Woman,* edited by L. Rodgers Rose, 217–232. New York: Sage.

Gilkes, Cheryl T. 2001. *If It Wasn't for the Women: Black Women's Experience and Womanist Culture in Church and Community.* Maryknoll: Orbis Books.

Gillham, Bill. 2005. *Research Interviewing: The Range of Techniques: A Practical Guide.* London: McGraw-Hill Education.

Glaser, Barney G., and Anselm L. Strauss. 1967. *Discovery of Grounded Theory: Strategies for Qualitative Research.* London: Routledge.

Goode, William J. 1959. "The Theoretical Importance of Love." *American Sociological Review* 24, no. 1: 38–47.

Goodwin, Jeff, & Jasper, James. 2006. "Emotions and Social Movements." In *Handbook of the Sociology of Emotions*, edited by Jan E. Stets and Jonathan H. Turner, 611–635. Boston: Springer Press.

Gould, Deborah B. 2009. *Moving Politics: Emotion and ACT UP's Fight against AIDS*. Chicago: University of Chicago Press.

Guest, Greg, Arwen Bunce, and Laura Johnson. 2006. "How Many Interviews Are Enough? An Experiment with Data Saturation and Variability." *Field Methods* 18, no. 1: 59–82.

Halkitis, Perry N., Sandra A. Kupprat, and Preetika Pandey Mukherjee. 2010. "Longitudinal Associations between Case Management and Supportive Services Use among Black and Latina HIV-Positive Women in New York City." *Journal of Women's Health* 19, no. 1: 99–108.

Hamlet, Janice D. 2000. "Assessing Womanist Thought: The Rhetoric of Susan L. Taylor." *Communication Quarterly* 48, no. 4: 420–436.

Hammonds, Evelynn. 1995. "Missing Persons: African American Women, AIDS, and the History of Disease." In *Words of Fire: An Anthology of African American Feminist Thought,* edited by Beverly Guy-Sheftal, 434–449. New York: The New Press.

Harris, Angelique and Bartlow, Susannah. 2015. "Intersectionality: Race, Gender, Sexuality, and Class." In *Handbook of the Sociology of Sexualities,* edited by John DeLamater and Rebecca Plante, 261–271. Boston: Springer Press.

Harris, Angelique. 2010. "AIDS Promotion within the Black Church: Social Marketing in Action." *Social Marketing Quarterly* 16, no. 4: 71–91.

Harris, Melanie L. 2017. *Ecowomanism: African American Women and Earth-Honoring Faiths*. Maryknoll Orbis Books.

Hayes, Diana L. 2016. *No Crystal Stair: Womanist Spirituality*. Maryknoll: Orbis Books.

Herek, Gregory M., and John P. Capitanio. 1999. "AIDS Stigma and Sexual Prejudice." *American Behavioral Scientist* 42, no. 7: 1130–1147.

Hochschild, Arlie Russell. 1979. "Emotion Work, Feeling Rules, and Social Structure." *American Journal of Sociology* 85, no. 3: 551–575.

Hochschild, Arlie Russell. 1983. The Managed Hearts: The Commercialization of Human Emotion. Berkeley: University of California Press.

Hochschild, Arlie Russell. 2003. *The Second Shift*. New York: Penguin Books.

Hochschild, Arlie Russell. 2010. "The Managed Heart: Commercialization of Human Feeling." In *The Production of Reality: Essays and Readings on Social Interaction*, edited by Jodi O'Brian, 320–336. Thousand Oaks: Sage Publications.

Hoffman, Nancy. 1986. "Teaching about Slavery, the Abolitionist Movement, and Women's Suffrage." *Women's Studies Quarterly* 14, no1/2: 2–6.

Hoggett, Paul. 2015. *Politics, Identity, and Emotion*. London: Routledge.

hooks, bell. 1981. *Ain't I A Woman: Black Women and Feminism*. London: Routledge.

Hoosen, Sarah, and Anthony Collins. 2004. "Sex, Sexuality and Sickness: Discourses of Gender and HIV/AIDS among KwaZulu-Natal Women." *South African Journal of Psychology* 34, no. 3: 487–505.

Hudson-Weems, Clenora. 2019: *Africana Womanism: Reclaiming Ourselves*. London: Routledge.

Hurston, Zora Neale, Mary Helen Washington, and Henry Louis, Jr. 1937. *Their Eyes Were Watching God: A Novel*. Westport: Greenwood Press.

Ingram, Deborah, and Sally A. Hutchinson. 2000. "Double Binds and the Reproductive and Mothering Experiences of HIV-Positive Women." *Qualitative Health Research* 10, no. 1: 117–132.

Jain, Vardhmaan, Mahmoud Al Rifai, Michelle T. Lee, Ankur Kalra, Laura A. Petersen, Elizabeth M. Vaughan, Nathan D. Wong, Christie M. Ballantyne, and Salim S. Virani. 2021. "Racial and Geographic Disparities in Internet Use in the US among Patients with Hypertension or Diabetes: Implications for Telehealth in the Era of COVID-19." *Diabetes Care* 44, no. 1: e15-e17.

Jenkins, J. Craig. 1983. "Resource Mobilization Theory and the Study of Social Movements." *Annual Review of Sociology* 9, no. 1: 527–553.

Johnson, Ernest H., Larry Gant, Yvonne A. Hinkle, Douglas Gilbert, Cassandra Willis, and Tanya Hoopwood. 1992. "Do African-American Men and Women Differ in Their Knowledge about AIDS, Attitudes about Condoms, and Sexual Behaviors?" *Journal of the National Medical Association* 84, no. 1: 9–64.

Johnson, Mark. 2013. *The Body in the Mind: The Bodily Basis of Meaning, Imagination, and Reason*. Chicago: University of Chicago Press.

Kaba, Mariame. 2021. *We Do This 'Til We Free Us: Abolitionist Organizing and Transforming Justice*. Chicago: Haymarket Books.

Kemper, Theodore D. 1987. "How Many Emotions Are There? Wedding the Social and the Autonomic Components." *American Journal of Sociology* 93, no. 2: 263–289.

Khaleeli, Homa. 2021. "#SayHerName: Why Kimberlé Crenshaw Is Fighting for Forgotten Women." The Guardian. Last modified May 30, 2016. https://www .theguardian.com/lifeandstyle/2016/may/30/sayhername-why-kimberle-crenshaw -is-fighting-for-forgotten-women.

King, James L., and Karen Hunter. 2004. *On the Down Low: A Journey into the Lives of "Straight" Black Men Who Sleep with Men*. New York: Broadway Books.

Klonoff, Elizabeth A., and Hope Landrine. 1999. "Do Blacks Believe That HIV/AIDS Is a Government Conspiracy against Them?" *Preventive Medicine* 28, no. 5: 451–457.

Kornegay, E. L. 2004. "Queering Black Homophobia: Black Theology as a Sexual Discourse of Transformation." *Theology & Sexuality* 11, no. 1: 29–51.

Kvasny, Lynette, and Fay Cobb Payton. 2018. "Managing Hypervisibility in the HIV Prevention Information–Seeking Practices of Black Female College Students." *Journal of the Association for Information Science and Technology* 69, no. 6: 798–806.

Lightsey, Pamela. 2015. *Our Lives Matter: A Womanist Queer Theology*. Eugene: Wipf and Stock Publishers.

Lincoln, C. Eric, and Lawrence H. Mamiya. 1990. *The Black Church in the African American Experience*. Durham: Duke University Press.

The Nation. 2017. "Sexual Harassment Law Was Shaped by the Battles of Black Women: Their Stories Should Guide Us in Propelling the #MeToo Momentum Forward. https://www.thenation.com/article/archive/sexual-harassment-law-was -shaped-by-the-battles-of-black-women/.

Lorde, Audre. 1984a [1979]. *Sister Outsider: Essays and Speeches*. New York: Penguin Classics.

Lorde, Audre. 1984b [1979]. "The Master's Tools Will Never Dismantle the Master's House (Comments at the 'The Personal and the Political Panel')." In *Sister Outsider: Essays and Speeches*, 110–113. Toronto: Sister Visions Press.

Mackenzie, Sonja. 2013. *Structural Intimacies: Sexual Stories in the Black AIDS Epidemic*. Newark: Rutgers University Press.

Maparyan, Layli. 2012. *The Womanist Idea*. London: Routledge.

Marr, Vanessa Lynn. 2014. "Growing 'Homeplace': In Critical Service-Learning: An Urban Womanist Pedagogy." PhD diss., Wayne State University.

McDonald, Katrina Bell. 1997. "Black Activist Mothering: A Historical Intersection of Race, Gender, and Class." *Gender & Society* 11, no. 6: 773–795.

McDoom, M. Maya, Barbara Bokhour, Meg Sullivan, and Mari-Lynn Drainoni. 2015. "How Older Black Women Perceive the Effects of Stigma and Social Support on Engagement in HIV Care." *AIDS Patient Care and STDs* 29, no. 2: 95–101.

McLane-Davison, D. 2018. "The Art of Activist Mothering: Black Feminist Leadership & Knowing What to Do." *In What the Village Gave Me: Conceptualization of Womanhood*, edited by Denise Davis-Maye, Annice D. Yarber, Tonya E. Perry, 137–160. Lanham: University Press of America.

McLane-Davison, Denise. 2016. "Lifting: Black Feminist Leadership in the Fight against HIV/AIDS." *Affilia* 31, no. 1: 55–69.

Mercado, Carla, Gloria Beckles, Yiling Cheng, Kai McKeever Bullard, Sharon Saydah, Edward Gregg, and Giuseppina Imperatore. 2021. "Trends and Socioeconomic Disparities in All-Cause Mortality among Adults with Diagnosed Diabetes by Race/Ethnicity: A Population-Based Cohort Study-USA, 1997–2015." *British Medical Journal* 11, no. 5: e044158.

Millett, Gregorio, David Malebranche, Byron Mason, and Pilgrim Spikes. 2005. "Focusing 'Down Low': Bisexual Black Men, HIV Risk and Heterosexual Transmission." *Journal of the National Medical Association* 97, no. 7 Suppl: 52S-59S.

Morgen, Sandra. 2002. *Into Our Own Hands: The Women's Health Movement in the United States, 1969–1990*. Newark: Rutgers University Press.

Muvuka, Baraka, Ryan M. Combs, Suur D. Ayangeakaa, Nida M. Ali, Monica L. Wendel, and Trinidad Jackson. 2020. "Health Literacy in African-American Communities: Barriers and Strategies." *Health Literacy Research and Practice* 4, no. 3: e138-e143.

Newman, Peter A., Charmaine C. Williams, Notisha Massaquoi, Marsha Brown, and Carmen Logie. 2008. "HIV Prevention for Black Women: Structural Barriers and Opportunities." *Journal of Health Care for the Poor and Underserved* 19, no. 3: 829–841.

Nydegger, Liesl A., Julia Dickson-Gomez, and Thant Ko. 2021. "A Longitudinal, Qualitative Exploration of Perceived HIV Risk, Healthcare Experiences, and Social Support as Facilitators and Barriers to PrEP Adoption among Black Women." *AIDS and Behavior* 25, no. 2: 582–591.

Ogunyemi, Chikwenye Okonjo. 1985. "Womanism: The Dynamics of the Contemporary Black Female Novel in English." *Signs: Journal of Women in Culture and Society* 11, no. 1: 63–80.

Ojikutu, B. O., N. Amutah-Onukagha, T. F. Mahoney, C. Tibbitt, S. D. Dale, K. H. Mayer, and L. M. Bogart. 2020. "HIV-Related Mistrust (or HIV Conspiracy Theories) and Willingness to Use PrEP among Black Women in the United States." *AIDS and Behavior* 24, no. 10: 2927–2934.

Olson, Lynne. 2001. *Freedom's Daughters: The Unsung Heroines of the Civil Rights Movement from 1830 to 1970*. New York City: Simon and Schuster.

Patton, Cindy. 2005. *Last Served? Gendering the HIV Pandemic*. London: Taylor & Francis.

Pellerin, Marquita. 2012. "Defining Africana Womanhood: Developing an Africana Womanism Methodology." *Western Journal of Black Studies* 36, no. 1: 76–85.

Peterson, Gretchen. 2006. "Cultural Theory and Emotions." In *Handbook of the Sociology of Emotions*, edited by Jan E. Stets and Jonathan H. Turner, 114–134. Boston: Springer Press.

Pettaway, Lincoln, Lawrence Bryant, Florence Keane, and Shelley Craig. 2014. "Becoming Down Low: A Review of the Literature on Black Men Who Have Sex with Men and Women." *Journal of Bisexuality* 14, no. 2: 209–221.

Phillips, Layli. 2006. "The Womanist Reader: The First Quarter Century of Womanist Thought." London: Routledge.

Plutchik, Robert. 2003. *Emotions and Life: Perspectives from Psychology, Biology, and Evolution*. Washington DC: American Psychological Association.

Rayner, Brian L., and J. David Spence. 2021. "Physiological Treatment of Hypertension in Black Patients: Time for Action." *Circulation* 143, no. 34: 2367–2369.

Reed, Pamela Yaa Asantewaa. 2001. "Africana Womanism and African Feminism: A Philosophical, Literary, and Cosmological Dialectic on Family." *Western Journal of Black Studies* 25, no. 3: 168–176.

Reeder, Glenn D., Denise McLane Davison, Keshia L. Gipson, and Matthew S. Hesson-McInnis. 2001. "Identifying the Motivations of African American Volunteers Working to Prevent HIV/AIDS." *AIDS Education and Prevention* 13, no. 4: 343–354.

Richardson, Allissa V. 2019. "Dismantling Respectability: The Rise of New Womanist Communication Models in the Era of Black Lives Matter." *Journal of Communication* 69, no. 2: 193–213.

Rikard, R. V., Maxine S. Thompson, Rachel Head, Carlotta McNeil, and Caressa White. 2012. "Problem Posing and Cultural Tailoring: Developing an HIV/AIDS Health Literacy Toolkit with the African American Community." *Health Promotion Practice* 13, no. 5: 626–636.

Roberts, Dorothy E. 1999. *Killing the Black Body: Race, Reproduction, and the Meaning of Liberty*. London: Vintage Press.

Robins, Steven. 2006. "From 'Rights' to 'Ritual': AIDS Activism in South Africa." *American Anthropologist* 108, no. 2: 312–323.

Rosenberg, Morris. 1990. "Reflexivity and Emotions." *Social Psychology Quarterly* 53, no. 1: 3–12.

Rosenberg, Morris. 1991. "Self-Processes and Emotional Experiences." In *The Self-Society Interface: Cognition, Emotion, and Action*, edited by Judith Howard and Peter Callero, 123–142. New York: Cambridge University Press.

Saleh, Lena Denise, and Don Operario. 2009. "Moving Beyond "the Down Low": A Critical Analysis of Terminology Guiding HIV Prevention Efforts for African American Men Who Have Secretive Sex with Men." *Social Science & Medicine* 68, no. 2: 390–395.

Schachter, Stanley, and Jerome Singer. 1962. "Cognitive, Social, and Physiological Determinants of Emotional State." *Psychological Review* 69, no. 5: 379–399.

Schieman, Scott. 2006. "Anger." In *Handbook of the Sociology of Emotions*, edited by Jan E. Stets and Jonathan H. Turner, 493–515. Boston: Springer Books.

Seidman, Irving. 2006. *Interviewing as Qualitative Research: A Guide for Researchers in Education and the Social Sciences*. New York: Teachers College Press.

Shambley-Ebron, Donna Z., and Joyceen S. Boyle. 2006. "Self-Care and Mothering in African American Women with HIV/AIDS." *Western Journal of Nursing Research* 28, no. 1: 42–60.

Shields, Stephanie, Dallas Gerner, Brooke Di Leone, and Alina Hadley. 2006. "Gender and Emotion." In *Handbook of the Sociology of Emotions*, edited by Jan E. Stets and Jonathan H. Turner, 63–83. Boston, Springer Press.

Simons, Margaret. 1979. "Racism and Feminism: A Schism in the Sisterhood." *Feminist Studies* 5, no. 2: 384–401.

Smith, Justin, Emma Simmons, and Kenneth H. Mayer. 2005. "HIV/AIDS and the Black Church: What Are the Barriers to Prevention Services?" *Journal of the National Medical Association* 97, no. 12 (2005): 1682–1685.

Smith, Susan L. 1995. *Sick and Tired of Being Sick and Tired*. Pittsburg: University of Pennsylvania Press.

Smith-Ireland, Sheila. 2018. "How Do African-American Female Executives Maintain Their Authenticity as African-American Women in Executive Leadership Roles: A Generic Qualitative Inquiry." PhD diss., Capella University.

Springer, Kimberly. 2005. *Living for the Revolution: Black Feminist Organizations, 1968–1980*. Durham: Duke University Press.

Snow, David A., and Robert D. Benford. 1992. "Master Frames and Cycles of Protest." In *Frontiers in Social Movement Theory*, edited by Alson Morris and Carol Mueller, 133–156. New Haven: Yale University Press.

Stephens, Dionne P., and Layli D. Phillips. 2003. "Freaks, Gold Diggers, Divas, and Dykes: The Sociohistorical Development of Adolescent African American Women's Sexual Scripts." *Sexuality and Culture* 7, no. 1: 3–49.

Stephens, Dionne P., and April L. Few. 2007. "Hip Hop Honey or Video Ho: African American Preadolescents' Understanding of Female Sexual Scripts in Hip Hop Culture." *Sexuality & Culture* 11, no. 4: 48–69.

Stockdill, Brett C. 2003. *Activism against AIDS: At the Intersections of Sexuality, Race, Gender, and Class*. Boulder: Lynne Rienner Publisher.

Stoller, Nancy E. 1998. *Lessons from the Damned: Queers, Whores, and Junkies Respond to AIDS*. London: Routledge.

Sudbury, Julia. 2005. *"Other Kinds of Dreams": Black Women's Organizations and the Politics of Transformation.* London: Routledge.

Sutton, Madeline Y., and Carolyn P. Parks. 2013. "HIV/AIDS Prevention, Faith, and Spirituality among Black/African American and Latino Communities in the United States: Strengthening Scientific Faith-Based Efforts to Shift the Course of the Epidemic and Reduce HIV-Related Health Disparities." *Journal of Religion and Health* 52, no. 2: 514–530.

Sweet, Loretta S., and John B. Jemmott. 1991. "Applying the Theory of Reasoned Action to AIDS Risk Behavior: Condom Use among Black Women." *Nursing Research* 40, vol. 4: 228–34.

Taylor, Janette Y. 1998. "Womanism: A Methodologic Framework for African American Women." *Advances in Nursing Science* 21, no. 1: 53–64.

Taylor, Keeanga-Yamahtta. 2016. *From #BlackLivesMatter to Black Liberation.* Chicago: Haymarket Books.

Tharao, Wangari, Marvelous Muchenje, and Mira Mehes. 2013. "An Evidence-Based Intervention to Support African, Caribbean, and Black Women in Canada to Disclose Their HIV-Positive Status." In *Women and HIV Prevention in Canada: Implications for Research, Policy and Practice*, 105–134. London: Women's Press.

Thoits, Peggy A. 1989. "The Sociology of Emotions." *Annual Review of Sociology* 15, no. 1: 317–342.

Thomas, Stephen B., and Sandra Crouse Quinn. 1991. "The Tuskegee Syphilis Study, 1932 to 1972: Implications for HIV Education and AIDS Risk Education Programs in the Black Community." *American Journal of Public Health* 81, no. 11: 1498–1505.

Tilly, Charles. 2017 [1978]. *From Mobilization to Revolution.* London: Routledge.

Torrey, Jane W. 1979. "Racism and Feminism: Is Women's Liberation for Whites Only?" *Psychology of Women Quarterly* 4, no. 2: 281–293.

Townsend, Tiffany, Torsten Neilands, Anita Jones Thomas, and Tiffany. R. Jackson. 2010. "I'm No Jezebel; I Am Young, Gifted, and Black: Identity, Sexuality, and Black girls. *Psychology of Women Quarterly* 34(3): 273–285.

Vyavaharkar, Medha, Linda Moneyham, Sara Corwin, Ruth Saunders, Lucy Annang, and Abbas Tavakoli. 2010. "Relationships between Stigma, Social Support, and Depression in HIV-Infected African American Women Living in the Rural Southeastern United States." *Journal of the Association of Nurses in AIDS Care* 21, no. 2: 144–152.

Wagstaff, David A., Jeffrey A. Kelly, Melissa J. Perry, Kathleen J. Sikkema, Laura J. Solomon, Timothy G. Heckman, Eileen S. Anderson, and Community Housing AIDS Prevention Study Group. 1995. "Multiple Partners, Risky Partners and HIV Risk among Low-Income Urban Women." *Family Planning Perspectives* 27, no. 6: 241–245.

Walker, Alice. 1994. *In Search of Our Mothers' Gardens.* Durham: Duke University Press,

Walker-Barnes, Chanequa. 2014. Too Heavy a Yoke: Black Women and the Burden of Strength. Eugene: Cascade Books.

Washington, Harriet A. 2006. *Medical Apartheid: The Dark History of Medical Experimentation on Black Americans from Colonial Times to the Present.* New York: Doubleday Books.

Washington Post and The Kaiser Family Foundation. 2012. "*Washington Post*–Kaiser Family Foundation Poll of Black Women in America." *Washington Post.* Last modified February 12, 2012. http://www.washingtonpost.com/wp-srv/special /nation/black- women-in-america/.

Watkins-Hayes, Celeste. 2014. "Intersectionality and the Sociology of HIV/AIDS: Past, Present, and Future Research Directions." *Annual Review of Sociology* 40: 431–457.

Weisenfeld, Judith. 1997. *African American Women and Christian Activism: New York's Black YWCA, 1905–1945.* Cambridge: Harvard University Press.

Wells, Ida B. 2002. *On Lynchings.* Lanham: Rowman and Littlefield.

White, Deborah Gray. 1999. *Too Heavy a Load: Black Women in Defense of Themselves, 1894–1994.* New York: W. W. Norton & Company.

Whitmore, Suzanne K., Anna J. Satcher, and Sherry Hu. 2005. "Epidemiology of HIV/AIDS among Non-Hispanic Black Women in the United States." *Journal of the National Medical Association* 97, no. 7 Suppl: 19S-24S.

Williams, Carmen Braun. 2000. "African American Women, Afrocentrism and Feminism: Implications for Therapy." *Women & Therapy* 22, no. 4: 1–16.

Williams, Dolores S. 2013. *Sisters in the Wilderness: The Challenge of Womanist God-Talk.* Maryknoll: Orbis Books.

Wilson, Linette C. 2000. "Implementation and Evaluation of Church-Based Health Fairs." *Journal of Community Health Nursing* 17, no. 1: 39–48.

Wingood, Gina M., and Ralph J. DiClemente. 1998. "Partner Influences and Gender–Related Factors Associated with Noncondom Use among Young Adult African American Women." *American Journal of Community Psychology* 26, no. 1: 29–51.

Witt, Judith LaBorde. 1994. "The Gendered Division of Labor in Parental Caretaking: Biology or Socialization?" *Journal of Women & Aging* 6, no. 1–2: 65–89.

Wolcott, Victoria W. 2013. *Remaking Respectability: African American Women in Interwar Detroit.* Chappal Hill: UNC Press.

Wyatt, Gail Elizabeth, Jennifer Vargas Carmona, Tamra Burns Loeb, and John K. Williams. 2005. "HIV-Positive Black Women with Histories of Childhood Sexual Abuse: Patterns of Substance Use and Barriers to Health Care." *Journal of Health Care for the Poor and Underserved* 16, no. 4: 9–23.

Yancy, Clyde W. 2020. "COVID-19 and African Americans." *JAMA* 323, no. 19: 1891–1892.

Zahnd, Whitney E., Cathryn Murphy, Marie Knoll, Gabriel A. Benavidez, Kelsey R. Day, Radhika Ranganathan, Parthenia Luke et al. 2021. "The Intersection of Rural Residence and Minority Race/Ethnicity in Cancer Disparities in the United States." *International Journal of Environmental Research and Public Health* 18, no. 4: 1384.

Zinn, Maxine Baca, and Bonnie Thornton Dill. 2016. *Theorizing Difference from Multiracial Feminism.* London: Routledge.

Index

About the Authors

Dr. **Angelique Harris** is associate professor of medicine at Boston University and the director of faculty development and diversity in the Department of Medicine and director of faculty development at Boston University Medical Campus. Dr. Harris works to design, implement, and lead innovative programs and initiatives aimed at providing and promoting more equitable learning and working environments for faculty, staff, and students. An applied medical sociologist, Dr. Harris's research examines health, wellness, and resilience within marginalized communities and her areas of research expertise are in race and ethnicity, gender and sexualities, health and illness, social movements, cultural studies, and urban studies. More specifically, her research studies how groups construct health issues and how the marginalization and stigmatization they experience impact their access to resources and community mobilization.

Dr. **Omar Mushtaq** is lecturer at Chapman University. Dr. Mushtaq creates diversity and inclusion workshops and trainings for companies and organizations. Within sociology, his research areas include: health, race and ethnicity, gender and sexuality, and embodiment studies. His work explores the role that the intersections of race, gender, and sexuality have on sociocultural constructions of the body.

www.ingramcontent.com/pod-product-compliance
Lightning Source LLC
Chambersburg PA
CBHW021842290326
41932CB00064B/1210